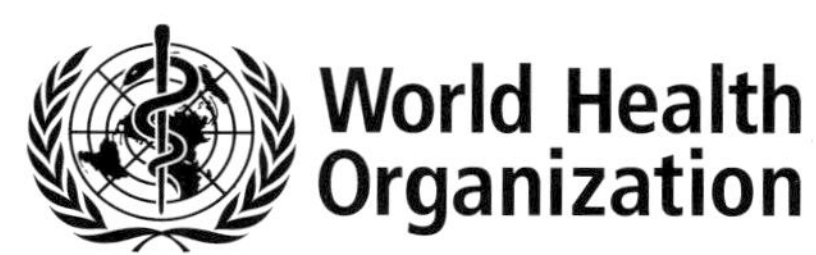

MEDICAL DEVICES: MANAGING THE MiSMatCh

An outcome of the Priority Medical Devices project

WHO Library Cataloguing-in-Publication Data

Medical devices: managing the mismatch: an outcome of the priority medical devices project.

1.Equipment and supplies - standards. 2.Cost of illness. 3.Biomedical engineering. 4.Research. 5.Appropriate technology. I.World Health Organization.

ISBN 978 92 4 156404 5   (NLM classification: WX 147)

Design & layout: L'IV Com Sàrl, Le Mont-sur-Lausanne, Switzerland.
Printed in France.

Contents

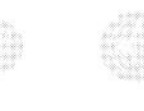

1. A stepwise approach to identifying gaps in medical devices
   (Availability Matrix and survey methodology)
2. Building bridges between diseases, disabilities and assistive devices:
   linking the GBD, ICF and ISO 9999
3. Clinical evidence for medical devices: regulatory processes focusing
   on Europe and the United States of America
4. Increasing complexity of medical devices and consequences
   for training and outcome of care
5. Context dependency of medical devices
6. Barriers to innovation in the field of medical devices
7. Trends in medical technology and expected impact on public health
8. Future public health needs: commonalities and differences
   between high- and low-resource settings

Boxes, figures and tables

Acknowledgements

The *Priority Medical Devices* project is the result of a collaboration, initiated in 2007, between the Dutch Ministry of Health, Welfare and Sport and the World Health Organization.

This publication was produced by the Department of Essential Health Technologies of the Health Systems and Services Cluster under the direction of Josée Hansen.

The project was supported by team coordinator Adriana Velazquez Berumen, Björn Fahlgren, Kaarina Klint, Kittie Rasmussen, Dima Samaha, Benjamin Schanker, Frederiek Swart, Gaby Vercauteren and Marieke Veurink. The preparation of this report would not have been possible without the support of the many colleagues at the World Health Organization headquarters and regional offices, including Steffen Groth, Director of the Department of Essential Health Technologies.

Thanks are due to Rhona MacDonald for writing and editing, John Maurice for writing, Dana Wickware for editing, Cathy Needham for copyediting, Kai Lashley for editing advice and proofreading, Rob Hoehn (Question Pro) for designing the Web survey, L'IV Com Sarl for layout and design, and Sue Hill for reviewing this report.

The support and guidance of the following experts, constituting the Steering Group, has been crucial to the development of the final report: David Banta, Mitchell D. Feldman, Adham Ismail, Carole Longson, Eric A. Mann, Les Olson, and Jeffrey A. Tice.

We wish to thank the following people for their contribution to the project: Fernao Beenkens, Pieter Stolk, Theo Bougie, Damian Carlson, Olugbenga Oyesanmi, Vivian Coates, Jonathan Gaev, Jenny Dankelman, Frank Painter, Yvonne Heerkens, Warren Kaplan, Annemiek Koster, Hristina Petkova, and Hans Werner.

Valuable inputs were received from the participants of Advisory Group meetings and the Informal consultation: Helen Alderson, Robby Bacchus, Joey A.M. Van Boxsel, Jie Chen, Francis Colardyn, Catherine Denis, Catherine Farrell, Lee T. Feldman, Chrystelle Gastaldi-Menager, Christian Hiesse, Maurice Hinsenkamp, Sabine Hoekstra, Robinah Kaitiritimba, Peter Leeflang, Bert Leufkens, Claude Manelfe, Utz P. Merten, Chiaki Miyoshi, Eoin O'Brien, Frank R. Painter, Agnette P. Peralta, Dulce Maria Martinez Pereira, Norberto Perico, M.S. Pillay, Tim Reed, Mahjoub Bashir Rishi, Michèle Roofe, Greg Shaw, Kunchala M. Shyamprasad, Henk Stam, Mariken Stoutmeijer, Per-Gunnar Svensson, Yot Teerawattananon, Ambrose Wasunna, Bart Wijnberg, David Williams, and Wim Wientjens.

For advice and support we are grateful to: Gerrit van Ark, Sube Banerjee, Arjan van Bergeijk, Saide Calil, Damian Carlson, Rens Damen, Adri Dumay, Renato Garcia, Jan H.B. Geertzen, Robert Geertsma, Michael Gropp, Hilbrand Haak, Hans Hofstraat, Kest Huijsman, Ann Keeling, Marijke de Kleijn - de Vrankrijker, Joy Lawn, Paul de Leeuw, Jan Meertens, Ahmed Meghzifene, Olugbenga Oyesanmi, Vikram Patel, Mark Perkins, Steve Plunkett, Roelf van Run, Frank Ruseler, Bas Streef, Peter Streef, Thijs Teeling, Jürgen Timm, Juan Esteban Valencia Zapata, Rex Widmer, Luc de Witte, and Jean Pierre Zellweger.

We would like to thank Gudrun Ingolfsdottir, Divina Maramba and Julia Miraillet for administrative support throughout the development of the report.

Photographs were provided by Caren Huygelen with the kind support of the following persons and institutions in the Netherlands: Academisch Medisch Centrum; B.L.M. Zijlmans, N.J. Reus, The Rotterdam Eye Hospital; Medisch Centrum Haaglanden, the Hague; Reinier de Graaf Groep, Delft; Vegro Verpleegartikelen, Katwijk (ZH); Universitair Medisch Centrum, Utrecht. Pictures were also provided by Maternal & Childhealth Advocacy International, United Kingdom, the World Health Organization, Geneva, Switzerland and UNAIDS, Geneva, Switzerland.

Acronyms and abbreviations

ACT	Artemesinin Combination Therapy
AGREE	Appraisal of Guidelines Research and Evaluation
AIDS	Acquired immunodeficiency syndrome
AMES	Assisted movement with enhanced sensation
BGSM	Blood glucose self-monitoring
CADTH	Canadian Agency for Drugs and Technologies in Health
CENETEC	National Center for Health Technology Excellence Mexico
COPD	Chronic obstructive pulmonary disease
CORDIS	European Commission's Community Research and Development Information Service
CT	Computerized axial tomography
DACEHTA	Danish Centre for Health Technology Assessment
DALY	Disability-adjusted life year
DFG	German Research Foundation
ECRI	Emergency Care Research Institute
ECG	Electrocardiogram
EU	European Union
EWH	Engineering World Health
FDA	United States Food and Drug Administration
GBD	Global burden of disease
GHTF	Global Harmonization Task Force
GMDN	Global Medical Device Nomenclature
HDI	Human Development Index
HIV	Human immunodeficiency virus
HTA	Health technology assessment
HRH	Human resources for health
ICD	International Classification of Diseases
ICF	International Classification of Functioning, Disability and Health
IDF	International Diabetes Federation
IHD	Ischaemic heart disease
IEC	International Electrotechnical Commission
IMPACT	International Medical Products Anti-Counterfeiting Taskforce
IMF	International Monetary Fund
IOL	Intraocular lens
ISO	International Organization for Standardization
ITU	International Telecommunication Union
LRTI	Lower respiratory tract infection
MHRA	Medicines and Healthcare products Regulatory Agency

MDI	Metered dose inhaler
MRI	Magnetic resonance imaging
NCAR	National Competent Authority Report programme
NICE	National Institute for Health and Clinical Excellence
NTD	Neglected tropical diseases
OECD	Organisation for Economic Co-operation and Development
PATH	[see: http://www.path.org for acronym]
PET	Positron emission tomography
PMD	Priority Medical Devices
PPP	Public-private-partnership
R&D	Research and development
RTA	Road Traffic Accidents
SACH	Solid ankle cushion heel
SBU	Swedish Council on health technology Assessment in Health Care
SME	Small and medium enterprise
SPECT	Single photon emission computed tomography
TB	Tuberculosis
UGSM	Urine glucose self-monitoring
UMDNS	Universal Medical Device Nomenclature System
UNICEF	United Nations Children's Fund
UV	Ultraviolet
WHO	World Health Organization
YLD	Years lived with disability

Overview

Medical devices are important to provide health care and to improve the health of individuals and populations. The World Health Organization (WHO) recognizes this. One of WHO's strategic objectives is to ensure improved access, quality and use of medical devices. Without medical devices, routine medical procedures—from bandaging a sprained ankle, to diagnosing HIV/AIDS or implanting an artificial hip—would be impossible. Concurrently, modern technology is producing an overwhelming abundance of medical devices at a rate that soon makes the latest device obsolete.

Key issues affecting progress include the extreme diversity of the medical device arena—diverse in terms of types of devices, degrees of complexity, applications, usage, users and categories and issues like the context dependency of medical devices and research in medical devices often not based on public health needs.

However, as a crucial component of health care, medical devices will be most effective when considered in the wider context of the complete health-care package necessary to address public health needs: prevention, clinical care (investigation, diagnosis, treatment and management, follow up, and rehabilitation) and access to appropriate health care. Therefore, rather than just focusing on the technological issues involved in medical devices, it is necessary to frame medical devices in another way—as an agenda to improve global access to appropriate medical devices. This agenda is composed of the crucial "4 As"—Availability, Accessibility, Appropriateness, and Affordability. These four components help to widen the scope of the medical device agenda so that it does not just focus on "upstream" innovation efforts but also on choosing which medical devices to procure in a rational way, responding to the needs, and in ensuring that they are used as effectively as possible to best improve health.

A medical device needs to be appropriate for the context or setting in which it is intended. Context in this sense refers to linking the correct medical device with its corresponding health need to maximize its effectiveness. However, almost all devices present in developing countries have been designed for use in industrialized countries. Up to three quarters of these devices do not function in their new settings and remain unused. Factors contributing to this are: lack of needs assessment, appropriate design, robust infrastructure, spare parts when devices break down, consumables, and a lack of information for procurement and maintenance, as well as trained health-care staff. These issues are part of a broader problem in many countries: the lack of a medical device management system.

Further hampering the situation is the fact that unfortunately, medical device innovation and activities around the choosing and using of medical devices are currently often not based on public health needs.

In order to help move forward the agenda to improve global access to appropriate medical devices, the *Priority Medical Devices (PMD)* project, convened by WHO, developed a health based approach to medical devices. The first step in this approach was to identify the most important health problems: on a global level this means using the global burden of disease and/or disease risk factor estimates *(1)*. The second step was to identify how health problems are best managed by referring to relevant clinical guidelines. And the third and final step was to link the results of the first two steps to produce a list of key medical devices that are needed for the management of the identified high-burden diseases, at a given health-care level and in a given context.

Using this step-wise approach, the *PMD* project identified the key medical devices involved in the treatment and management of the global high-burden diseases from relevant clinical guidelines. Of particular note was the almost complete absence of any mention of assistive products necessary to help improve functionality of people with these diseases.

Further literature searches and qualitative research helped to identify problems and challenges regarding the key areas in choosing and using medical devices, medical device innovation, and possible solutions to barriers.

Medical device innovation is driven largely by the need for better solutions and for greater technological capabilities, and also by promising ideas, scientific interest and economic concerns. In addition, medical device innovation is mainly targeted at high-resource countries. To better align medical device innovation with public health needs, increased funding and improved infrastructure is necessary. In addition, better networking among stakeholders may help.

Choosing a medical device is complex and requires a transparent process based on reason, evidence and assessment of prioritized public health needs. Poor choices lead to inappropriate use or non-use of medical devices and a waste of resources. Barriers to rational choosing of a medical device include fascination with technology, aggressive marketing, high costs and inadequate information about the device. Possible solutions include improving access to information for decision-making and increasing the role of the biomedical engineer or similar experts.

One of the main barriers to optimal use of a medical device is the mismatch between the design of the device and the context in which it is used. An additional problem is lack of proper device management both at government level and within health-care facilities. Lack of standardization can also seriously hamper the usability and integration of devices. Possible solutions include developing designs of medical devices to make them more appropriate for a specific context, and improved staff training in specific medical device use.

This report suggests how an agenda to improve access to appropriate medical devices could be devised from applying the crucial 4 components—Availability, Accessibility, Appropriateness, and Affordability, to the 15 global high-burden diseases and some cross-cutting issues. The results of this exercise suggest several areas of research necessary to help make medical devices more available, accessible, appropriate, and affordable.

Examples include: development of a kit containing simple and affordable technologies for measuring blood pressure, blood glucose and cholesterol levels, which could assess cardiovascular risk; developing portable, affordable spirometry equipment for accurate diagnosis and prognosis of chronic obstructive pulmonary disease (COPD) or asthma in low-resource settings; and the development of more appropriate hearing aids which could potentially help people with hearing impairments whatever their age or setting. An example of a key cross-cutting issue is the need to develop simple, affordable, and reliable sensitivity tests for bacterial and viral antigens. Such tests could replace culture systems to detect the presence of pathogens and effectively and efficiently help to diagnose many high-burden infections and neglected tropical diseases.

The *PMD* project applied the "4 A" questions (Is the medical device: Available? Accessible? Appropriate? Affordable?) to some examples of identified key medical devices to further explore the downstream issues associated with poor access to appropriate medical devices.

The *PMD* project hopes all players in the medical device arena can collectively use the findings of this report to help make public health a central focus of their activities, along with the work on policies, tools and innovations of the WHO Global Initiative for Health Technologies *(2)*.[1]

---

1   Also see https://www.who.int/medical_devices/initiatives/en/, accessed 19 July 2010.

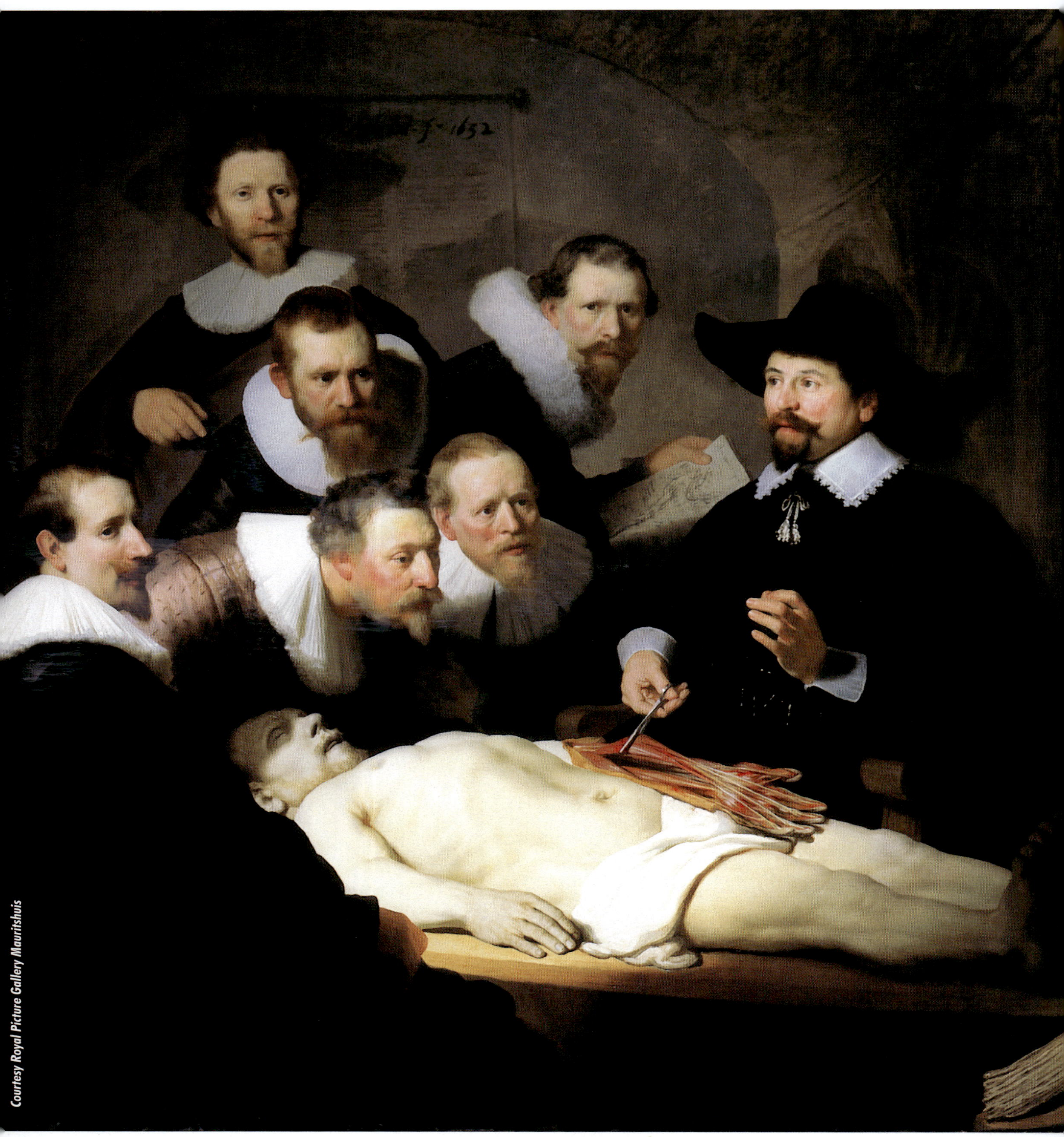

Introduction

For several centuries, people, mostly in high-resource settings, have benefited from a host of discoveries and developments that have improved health. The building of sewage and clean water systems, the discovery of pathogens and antibiotics, and the eradication of smallpox are notable examples.

In the medical device arena, outstanding developments to date have produced heart-lung machines and artificial joints, and the means to perform advanced brain surgery, to mention only a few examples. Modern medical technology (the application of medical devices) which dates its origins to the first half of the 19th century, only took off in earnest over the last 50 years. Very quickly, medical devices have become an essential part of health care and a vital component of the numerous activities carried out by health-care providers in their efforts to diagnose and treat people with medical conditions, and to alleviate the problems faced by people with functional disabilities.

Improvements in the health of many populations are associated with the improved ability to predict, prevent, diagnose and cure many illnesses, and to alleviate functioning problems using treatments and technologies that could hardly have been imagined a few decades ago. Among medical products commonly used in health care—such as medicines, vaccines and medical devices—the most abundant, diverse and widely used are medical devices. Reliable figures are lacking but widely accepted estimates put the number of different main categories of medical devices available on the world market today somewhere in the region of 10 000. Adding the vast number of different variants brings the figure to about 90 000 with some estimates putting the total as high as 1.5 million *(3)*.

Research is making rapid progress within the development of sophisticated medical technologies, such as genetic testing, genetic manipulation of living tissue, robotic surgery and remote patient management. Yet despite this progress, the majority of the world's population has little or no access to many of these innovations.

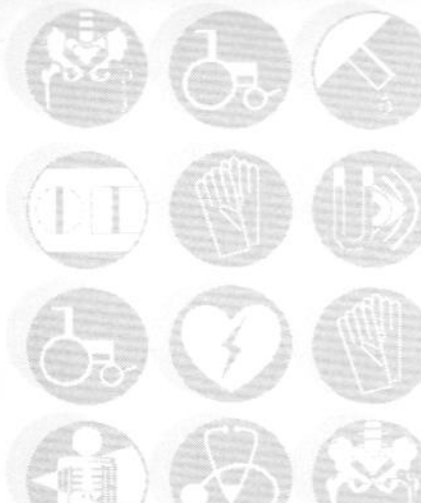

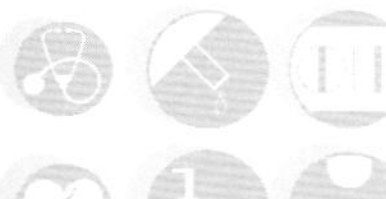

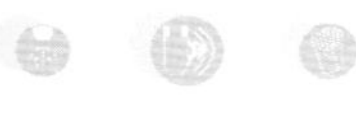
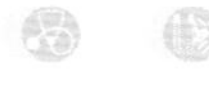

1.1 Prioritizing medical devices: setting the scene

Following the global impact of the landmark report *Priority medicines for Europe and the world (4)*—which proposed a specific research agenda leading to the creation of a public-private-partnership (PPP)—and the success of the 'access to essential medicines' agenda in focusing the attention of the international community on the specific needs, problems, and challenges of this crucial public health area, it is now time for the international community to focus on an agenda to improve access to appropriate medical devices that adequately addresses global public health needs. The concept of appropriate medical devices is relevant to high-, middle-, or low-income settings although each may be viewed from different ends of the spectrum. For example, the abundance of high-tech, actively marketed medical devices in high-income settings may mean that medical devices are chosen and used based on factors other than clinical and public health need. In low-income settings, medical devices may be available but not adapted to be effectively used in the local context; for example, they may not withstand hot and dusty climates or may not run on insufficient electricity supplies.

Although there are many similarities to the issues involved in prioritizing medicines and the 'access to essential medicines' agenda, accessing appropriate medical devices has its own set of unique problems and challenges that urgently need solutions. It is important to note that although a crucial component of health care, access to appropriate medical devices will be most effective when considered in the wider context of the complete health-care package necessary to address public health needs: prevention, clinical care (investigation, diagnosis, treatment and management, follow-up, and rehabilitation) and access to appropriate health care.

Priority needs for health care and research can differ widely between high- and low-resource countries. Patients in high-resource countries may have a growing need for improved drug-releasing (eluting) cardiac stents and labour saving technologies. Patients in low-resource countries may urgently need simple, robust, affordable diagnostic tools, as well as strong, flexible wheelchairs for use on uneven roads, high curbs and narrow entrances.

Low-resource countries often lack the funds and purchasing power to assess or address their many vital needs. Industry in high-resource settings typically has little interest in investing in proper needs assessment and in the required research and development of medical devices for low-resource countries that promise a low return on that investment *(5)*.

These divergent priority needs are amplified by the fact that medical technology readily used in high-resource countries is often difficult or impossible to use in low-resource settings for lack of appropriate infrastructure, inappropriate design, lack of specialized human resources, to mention a few factors.

Medical research priorities in most high-resource countries are based primarily on scientific and technological preferences, with little explicit regard for public health needs *(6)*. In consequence, information about medical conditions and diseases does not translate into effective management of local health systems, nor does it translate into efforts to build the capability of low-resource countries to conduct and use research and to become technology innovators themselves.

Biomedical research contributes to scientific progress, to finding solutions to health problems, and to development, equity, global security and the fight against poverty *(7)*. As with similar health research areas, research relating to medical devices is not targeting populations in large parts of the world *(8)*. Most research activities focus on the needs of the industrialized countries.

Research pertinent to the needs of developing countries is "grossly under-resourced in many areas", according to the Global Forum on Health Research.[1] This discrepancy in health research funding is captured in the so-called "10/90 gap", a term coined in 1990 by the Global Forum on Health Research to highlight the fact that only 10% of global health research expenditure is devoted

---

[1] http://www.globalforumhealth.org/About/10-90-gap (accessed 17 July 2010).

to conditions that together account for 90% of the global disease burden *(9)*. Compounding the issue in many low-resource countries is the tendency for much of public health research spending—and of research agenda setting—to be concentrated under the control of academic centres in industrialized countries. Ideally, health research agendas should be national governments' responsibility. *The Priority Medical Devices (PMD)* project was established to help to address these problems.

1.2 The Priority Medical Devices project

In May 2007, the Sixtieth World Health Assembly expressed concern about the waste of resources resulting from inappropriate investments in health technologies—in particular, medical devices that do not meet high-priority needs, are incompatible with existing infrastructures, are irrationally or incorrectly used, or do not function efficiently. The World Health Assembly adopted resolution WHA60.29 and acknowledged the need "to contain burgeoning costs by establishing priorities in the selection and acquisition of health technologies … on the basis of their impact on the burden of disease, and to ensure the effective use of resources through proper planning, assessment, acquisition and management" *(10)*.

A strategic objective in the World Health Organization (WHO) plan for 2008–2013 *(11)* is to ensure improved access, quality and use of medical products including medical devices, thereby recognizing medical devices as a tool to provide health care and improve the health of people.

In 2007, with the support of the Ministry of Health, Welfare and Sport of the Netherlands, WHO established the *PMD* project to determine whether medical devices currently on the global market are meeting the needs of health-care providers and patients throughout the world and, if not, to propose remedial action based on sound research. The *PMD* project aimed at identifying gaps in the availability of medical devices and obstacles that might be hindering the full use of medical devices as public health tools. A second objective was the development of a methodology for identifying the medical devices needed to meet global public health needs. A third objective was to propose a possible research agenda for exploring how the gaps could be resolved and the obstacles removed.

As the project progressed, however, the following findings suggested that a change in the original objective of the project was necessary: 1) there are many medical devices available but not the most appropriate ones; 2) there are few gaps in the availability of medical devices on the market. These unanticipated findings prompted a project shift in focus to the many shortcomings related to medical devices. These problems, challenges, and failures amount to a mismatch, rather than a gap, that prevents medical devices from achieving their full public health potential.

1.3 The mismatch

In effect, the mismatch referred to above relates to medical devices coming to, and being available on, the market and the public health sector (i.e. that are accessible, affordable, and appropriate). Currently, there is no effective counter-force to absorb the large numbers of medical devices coming to the market and many factors contribute to this inadequate situation.

Industry may be capable of supplying the medical devices the world needs to promote health, prevent, diagnose, treat, and manage medical conditions and diseases, and alleviate functioning problems of people with disabilities. But the landscape is often cluttered with medical devices that have been acquired unnecessarily or irrationally, that are not being used safely and effectively for their intended purposes or even at all, and that, in too many cases, have not been adequately assessed for specific health outcomes.

One consequence of this mismatch is an inequity between the complex products of modern technological progress designed primarily for use in countries with adequate resources and infrastructure, and the relative paucity of medical devices specifically designed to be sufficiently robust and affordable for use in low-resource settings.

The mismatch will only be resolved when a countervailing force exists to focus the medical device market towards public health considerations at all stages of the medical device life-cycle. If this objective is to be achieved, the know-how, ingenuity and drive of the medical device industry will need to consider the quest for an equitable and cost-effective use of public health resources throughout the world.

1.4 This report

There are many steps along the path to successfully devising and achieving an agenda to improve global access to appropriate medical devices, and the main components involved are the crucial 4 As—Availability, Accessibility, Appropriateness, and Affordability. The initial work of the *PMD* project mostly took an "upstream" perspective, focusing on the activities involving manufacturers, such as innovation and research and development. However, given the importance of the "downstream" factors in successfully achieving global access to appropriate medical devices, this report also covers the downstream factors and includes the perspectives of potential buyers and users of medical devices.

This report has two objectives which align with the objectives of the *PMD* project. The first is to inform national health policy-makers, international organizations, manufacturers and other stakeholders(including users of medical devices) of the factors preventing the current medical device community from achieving its full public health potential. The second objective is to provide a basis on which all players on the medical device scene can, together, use the findings of this report to help make public health the central focus of their activities.

This report explores the medical device mismatch by analysing the two key issues involved in this disparity: 1) medical devices and 2) identifying and prioritizing public health needs. To help understand the issues involved, the report makes reference to the prioritizing medicines agenda, as the concepts involved in 'access to essential medicines' are already well known and can also be applied to the topic of global appropriate (i.e. context specific) medical devices. However, there are also some important differences that this report highlights.

The research components of the fact-finding remit of the project are documented in this report, and the issues raised are discussed in detail. This research involved:

1. Clinical guideline analysis to identify the key medical devices and assistive products associated with the 15 medical conditions and diseases contributing to the high-burden diseases globally.

2. Literature searches and specifically designed, and validated questionnaires to a) identify any clinical problems associated with the medical devices recommended for each high-burden medical condition (and suggest some further clinical research questions that may need to be addressed); b) identify the evidence base for, and past experience of, choosing and using medical devices, as well as for targeted medical device innovation; and c) identify possible ways of overcoming the barriers discovered.

Barriers to using and choosing medical devices and medical device innovation and possible ways to overcome these problems are discussed in detail in the *Medical devices: problems and possible solutions* section. To best illustrate the real situation in many countries, questions regarding the crucial 4 components—Availability, Accessibility, Appropriateness, and Affordability are applied to some examples of key medical devices.

The final section of the report describes a scoping exercise that brings together all the information and findings in the preceding sections to show how research options outlining potential access to appropriate medical devices can be devised from applying the crucial 4 components—Availability, Accessibility, Appropriateness, and Affordability, to the 15 diseases with the high-burden globally, risk factors, and cross-cutting themes. This exercise has the advantage of including the areas of research required for both the upstream (e.g. necessary clinical innovation), and downstream factors (e.g. technological research needed to make current medical devices more appropriate for low-income settings). Research into all of these areas is required to make the public health priority of global access to appropriate medical devices a reality.

There are many steps along the path to successfully devising and achieving an agenda to improve global access to appropriate medical devices, and the main components involved are the crucial 4 As—Availability, Accessibility, Appropriateness, and Affordability.

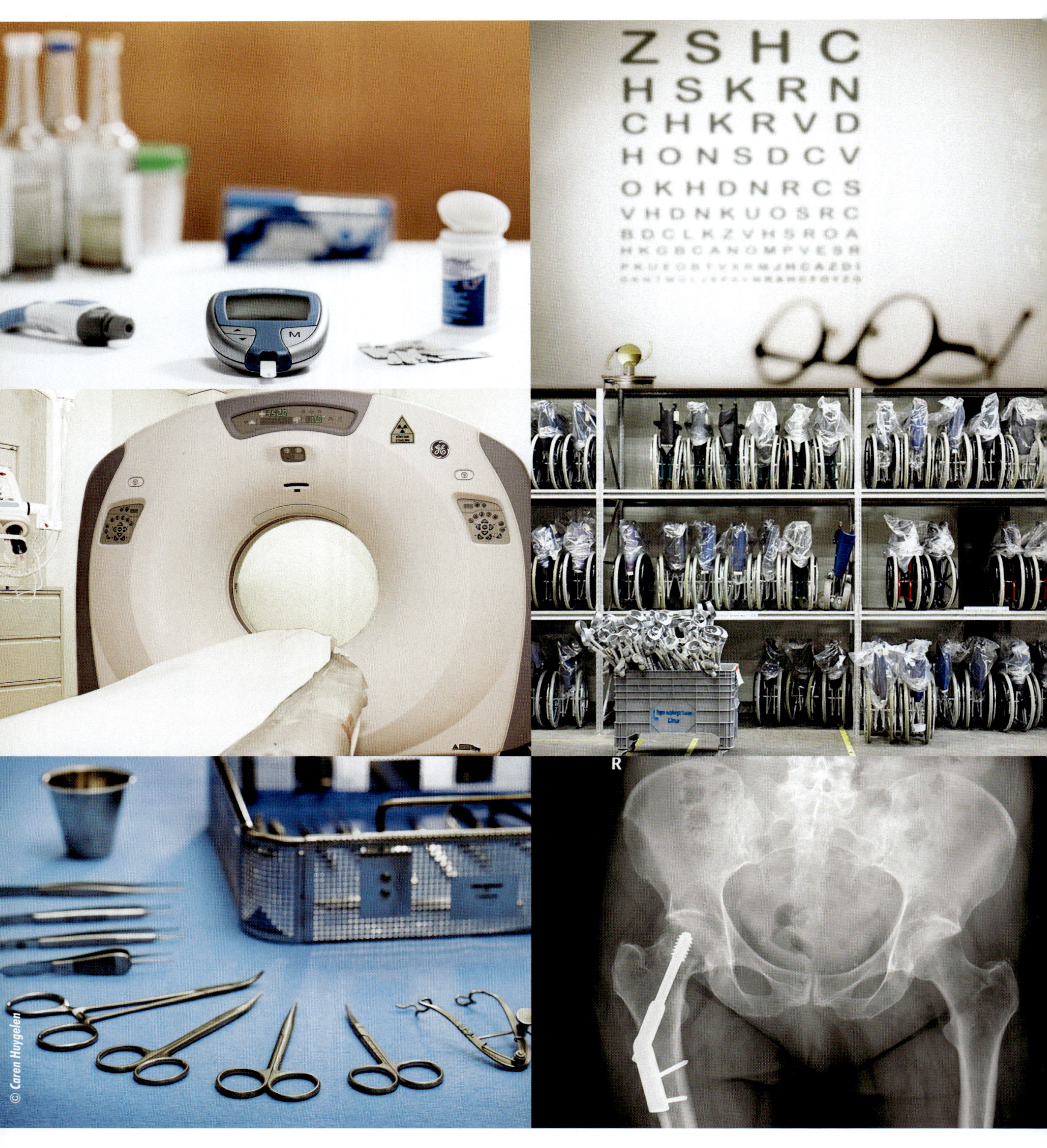

Z S H C
H S K R N
C H K R V D
H O N S D C V
O K H D N R C S
V H D N K U O S R C
B D C L K Z V H S R O A
H K G B C A N O M P V E S R
R

Medical devices

This section defines medical devices, gives a brief history, and highlights the similarities and differences between medical devices and medicines. Also included in this section is a description of the main areas involved in the medical device landscape that are crucial to the agenda to improve access of appropriate medical devices—supply, regulation and innovation. All three of these areas affect and influence the availability, accessibility, appropriateness, and affordability of medical devices. We refer to each of these four crucial components as they relate to the access to appropriate medical devices as follows:

Availability: in the context of this report is when a medical device can be found on the medical device market.

Accessibility: refers to people's ability to obtain and appropriately use good quality health technologies when they are needed.

Appropriate(ness): refers to medical methods, procedures, techniques, and equipment that are scientifically valid, adapted to local needs, acceptable to both patient and health-care personnel, and that can be utilized and maintained with resources the community or country can afford.

Affordability: the extent to which the intended clients of a health service or product can pay for it.

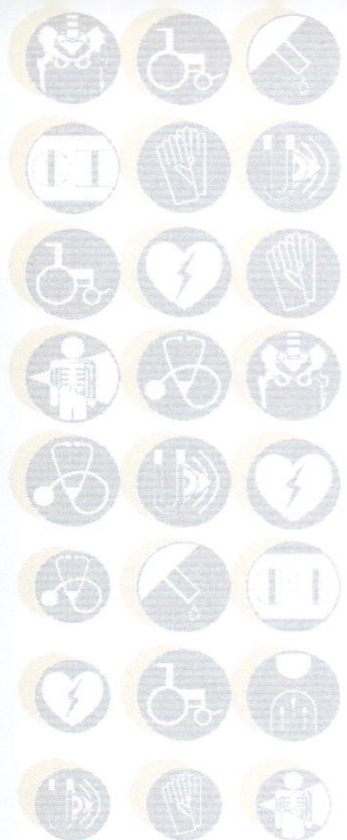

2.1 Medical devices: what's in a name?

Defining what is—and what is not—a medical device has never been easy. One reason is the multiplicity and diversity of devices. Another is the increasing number of products straddling the borderline between a device and a drug: a syringe prefilled with a medicinal product and a catheter coated with heparin to prevent blood clotting are two examples. Several countries and organizations have formulated a variety of definitions of a medical device. As the geographical span of trade in these devices has grown ever-more global and with it the need for regulatory control, so has the need for a single harmonized definition. In 2005, the Global Harmonization Task Force (GHTF), an expert group set up in 1992 jointly by regulatory authorities and the medical device industry, adopted a definition *(12)* that reflects the multitude of forms and uses of medical devices and that has since achieved wide acceptance.

The GHTF definition states, in summary,[1] that a medical device is any instrument, apparatus, implement, machine, appliance, implant, in vitro reagent or calibrator, software, material or other similar or related article that does not achieve its primary intended action in or on the human body solely by pharmacological, immunological or metabolic means and that is intended for human beings for:

- the diagnosis, prevention, monitoring, treatment or alleviation of disease;
- the diagnosis, monitoring, treatment, alleviation of, or compensation for an injury;
- the investigation, replacement, modification, or support of the anatomy or of a physiological process;
- supporting or sustaining life;
- controlling conception;
- disinfecting medical devices; and
- providing information for medical or diagnostic purposes by means of in vitro examination of specimens derived from the human body.

---

1   For the full definition of medical devices see *(12)*.

Box 2.1 Landmarks in medical device development

Sources: *(13–15)*.

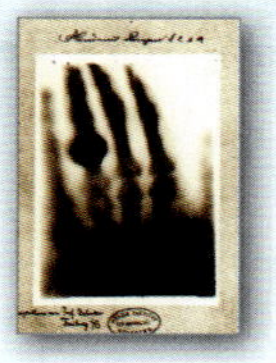

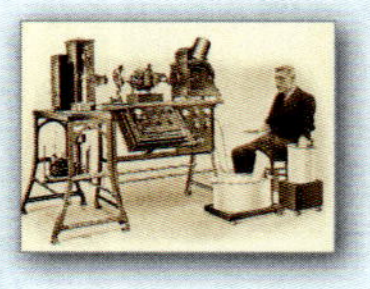

1903
FIRST ELECTROCARDIOGRAPH
Developed by Dutch physician and physiologist Willem Einthoven (awarded the Nobel Prize in 1924 for his discovery)

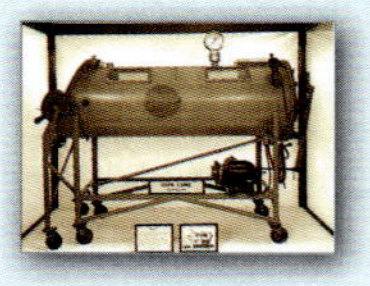

1927
FIRST MODERN RESPIRATOR
Devised by United States medical researcher Philip Drinker and his colleagues at Harvard University

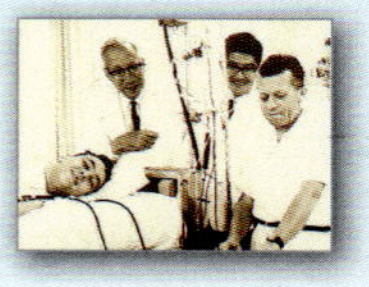

1945
FIRST KIDNEY DIALYSIS MACHINE
Invented by Dutch-born physician Willem Kolff

1890   1900   1910   1920   1930   1940

1800–1850
FIRST "MODERN" STETHOSCOPES, LARYNGOSCOPES, OPTHALMOSCOPES

1895
X-RAYS
Discovered by German physicist Wilhelm Roentgen

1928
FIRST CARDIAC CATHETERIZATION
Performed by Werner Forssmann on himself to show feasibility of technique for injecting drugs directly into the heart (co-recipient of the Nobel Prize in Physiology or Medicine in 1956)

1940
FIRST METALLIC HIP REPLACEMENT SURGERY
performed by United States surgeon Dr Austin T. Moore

Therefore, the GHTF definition of a "medical device" covers a multitude of different products. Some are complex and reflect the latest advances in technological progress: imaging equipment, lab-on-a-chip technology, and implants, for example. Most are relatively simple: tongue depressors, thermometers, stethoscopes, scales, latex gloves, sphygmomanometers, wound dressings, hospital beds, and crutches, to mention a few. Medical devices are essential to the successful delivery of almost every form of everyday health care, in every hospital, health-care centre, physician's office, ambulance and laboratory in every country, district and town.

Relatively basic procedures require a multitude of devices. For example, an appendectomy or childbirth can require devices including in vitro diagnostic tests, a hospital bed, surgical lamps, drapes, surgical instruments, an operating room table, surgical gloves and masks, syringes, infusion sets, dressings, gauze swabs, emesis basins, a speculum, to mention only a few. But even the more complex procedures, such as organ transplants, neurosurgery and cardiac valve replacement also require many of the above-mentioned medical devices; in fact they are required for just about every form of health care.

2.2 Past, present, and future

Medical devices have been in existence for centuries. There is evidence that scalpels, slings, splints, crutches and other medical devices were used as far back as 7000 BCE by the Egyptians. Box 2.1 shows the landmarks and key trends in more recent medical device development.

2.2.1 Recent key trends

1980s: Surge in the number of patient care medical devices, particularly high-resolution imaging

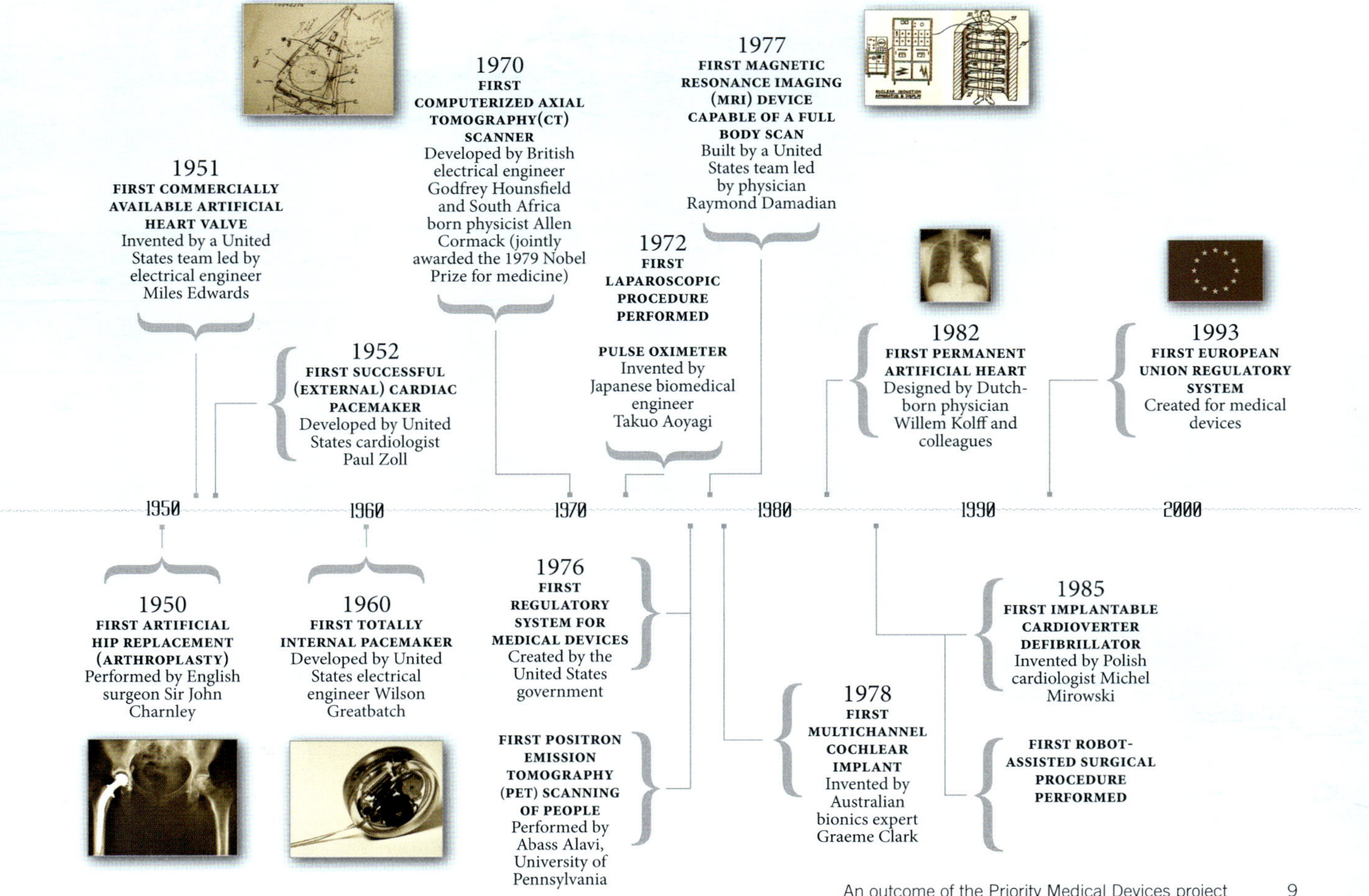

devices, notably radiographic and fluoroscopic units. Systems for continuous monitoring of cardiovascular parameters—heart rate, heart output and blood pressure—were becoming standard hospital fixtures. Treatment was taken over by technological progress—ventilators, kidney dialysis machines and neonatal incubators were becoming commonplace *(16)*.

1980s to 2000: Most hospitals in industrialized countries adopted computerized axial tomography (CT) scanners and magnetic resonance imaging (MRI) units. Surgeons, too, could offer their patients a growing list of medical devices to replace body parts. Choice of medical devices grew exponentially *(17)*.

2000–10: Robotics became a reality of the medical device world with proponents and opponents *(18)*. The choices of assistive devices to people with functional disabilities rose dramatically and the concept of medical devices integrated with information systems

or web-based system exploded. This integration has several advantages but also some disadvantages *(18–23)*.

2.2.2 Future trends

Smaller and less expensive robotic systems that allow high-precision surgery will continue to be developed, notably for orthopaedic and neurological procedures. Synergy and miniaturization will direct future innovation in medical device design, such as "smart medical capsules" *(18, 24, 25)*. Nanotechnology and genomics will interact to continue the rise in personalized care. Tissue-engineered products will continue to emerge from the convergence of different health care-related disciplines, such as the biological sciences, nanotechnology, cognitive sciences, information technology and material science *(26, 27)*.

The lure of technology is strong, but the cost-effectiveness, real need, and likely usefulness of

---

Box 2.2 Implications of technology trends

Three current trends which are likely to have a significant effect on the use of medical devices and their expected health implications.

Technology convergence
Medical device implications
- labour-intensive, costly and requiring multi-disciplinary teams
- highly dependent on infrastructure and therefore difficult to apply in low-resource settings
- likely to raise patient expectations and patient pressure on health care
- likely to be reserved for financially privileged patients
- liable to incur technical risks and patient safety problems

Health implications
- could enhance sharing of clinical information
- could reduce errors of data entry and facilitate data analysis
- could enhance clinician efficiency and allow increased case load
- could improve patient outcomes and patient safety by giving clinicians access to all patient data

Decentralization of care delivery
Medical device implications
- reliance on portable devices, which would require greater ruggedness than stationary hospital equipment
- reliance on non-medical technology (e.g. communication networks, durable battery technology, and power sources)

Health implications
- benefit to patients and family caregivers, but would require

adequate user training
- more patients receiving care outside the hospital setting
- patient monitoring more efficient and health care more timely
- enables access of rural health-care professionals to highly specialized clinical procedures

Computer-aided surgery and robotics
Medical device implications
- risk of use error or malfunctioning of the system and consequent patient injury
- longer learning curve for users
- requires integration of imaging and surgical navigation systems
- device-specific training required
- high acquisition and procedure costs that could be prohibitive for many resource-scarce settings
- maintenance and quality control requirements likely to be demanding

Health implications
- greater accuracy of surgical procedures
- time-saving (despite long initial learning curve)
- greater consistency and reproduction of procedures
- could circumvent obstacles to surgical intervention (such as unusual anatomy and poor visibility of target tissue)
- allows frequent checking of instrument status and positioning
- could give nurses more time with patients by alleviating menial tasks.

Source: *(31)*.

many innovative technologies are questionable. For example ultrahigh-field-strength MRIs, robotic-assisted surgical systems, and proton radiation therapy have uncertain benefits and high financial costs *(28, 29)*.

Another example is a growing trend among medical imaging facilities is to promote "whole-body" CT scanning as a preventive measure for people who have no symptoms and no suspected disease. In July 2009, the United States Food and Drug Administration (FDA) announced that it "has never approved or cleared or certified any CT system specifically for use in screening, because no manufacturer has ever demonstrated to the FDA that their CT scanner is effective for screening for any disease or condition". Furthermore, the FDA warned of the risk of radiation doses through repetitive CT examination *(30)*.

In addition, devices are increasingly used sequentially or simultaneously to achieve a specific health outcome. A common example is the insertion of a coronary stent, which calls for using numerous tools to select appropriate patients, complete the procedure and follow-up, including electrocardiography, angiography, ultrasound, and anticoagulation therapy.

Another cross-cutting technology trend is the convergence of different health care-related disciplines, such as the biological sciences, nanotechnology, cognitive sciences, information technology, and material science *(26, 27)*. Box 2.2 highlights the implications of these trends in medical device technology.

2.3 Assistive products

Assistive products deserve a special mention as they are intrinsically involved in helping to overcome functioning problems relating to disability. Assistive products are generally not related to medical diagnosis but to problems with functioning. They are used to maintain or enhance functioning and minimize disability of the person using them, rather than to cure a disease or condition *(32)*. In 2005, the Fifty-eighth World Health Assembly called on WHO and its Member States to facilitate the development

of, and improve access to, assistive products *(33)*. Assistive products and technologies such as wheelchairs, prostheses, mobility aids, hearing aids, visual aids, and specialized computer software and hardware can help to improve functionality and restore social inclusion.

Assistive products needed by a patient to improve functioning are classified by the International classification of assistive products for persons with disability, the ISO 9999.[2] ISO 9999 is the international standard that establishes a classification of assistive products for persons with disabilities. The most recent version is the one published in 2007 *(34)*.[3] The definition of an assistive product according to the ISO 9999 (2007):

"An assistive product is any product (including devices, equipment, instruments, technology and software) especially produced or generally available, for preventing, compensating, monitoring, relieving or neutralizing impairments, activity limitations and participation restrictions."

In November 2009, Working Group ISO TC173/SC2/WG 11[4] agreed upon a slightly adapted version:[5]
* An assistive product is any product (including devices, equipment, instruments and software) especially produced or generally available, used by or for persons with disability
  * for participation;
  * to protect, support, train, measure or substitute for body functions/structures and activities; or
  * to prevent impairments, activity limitations or participation restrictions.

The choice of assistive products to help people with functional disabilities has grown. Examples of such "assistive" technology *(35)* include:
* Mobility aids—wheelchairs, powered scooters, walking aids, artificial limbs;
* Environmental assistive devices (also known as

---

2   Medical devices according to the definition of the GHTF and assistive products according to ISO 9999 partly overlap. In ISO 9999 (Assistive products for persons with disability – Classification and terminology), the term "assistive products" is used instead of assistive medical devices. Many but not all of the assistive products are assistive medical devices.

3   ISO is the abbreviation of the International Organization for Standardization. The ISO 9999 is controlled and updated by ISOs Subcommittee 2 (responsible for classification and terminology) of Technical Committee 173 (responsible for assistive products for persons with disability).

4   Working Group ISO TC 173/SC2/wg 11 consists of international experts involved in the continuous revision process of ISO 9999.

5   This definition is included in the Draft International Standard (DIS) of ISO 9999 – version 2011, published in February 2010.

ambient assisted living, domotics or telecare) that sense smoke, flooding, gas leaks and other hazards in the home, or remind people to take a medicine or that call for help if needed; remote control systems to open and close doors and windows, and to perform other common household tasks;
- Moving and handling systems—hoists, slider boards, bath lifts, stair lifts;
- Lingual speech synthesis and voice recognition software;
- Talking software browsers and software that converts text from a document or an e-mail message into audible speech; and
- Voice-activated telephone controls.

The danger, however, of designing a device, particularly an assistive device, for use by people with disabilities is that the user and the user's disability can become the object of social stigma. Hence the call by some observers for medical, particularly assistive, devices that offer a "universal, or inclusive", design that facilitates use by any user, whether he or she has any disabilities or not *(36)*.

2.4 Pharmaceuticals and medical devices: similarities and differences

Pharmaceuticals and medical devices are similar in certain aspects: both are health technologies, both can be used to diagnose, treat, alleviate, and cure disease, both require regulatory oversight and a post-market surveillance system, both have intellectual property issues, both need a supply chain and both have become an integral part of modern health care.

2.4.1 Access to essential medicines

The vision of the 'access to essential medicines' agenda *(37)* is that people everywhere have access to the essential medicines they need; that the medicines are safe, effective and of assured quality; and that they are prescribed and used rationally. Improved availability, accessibility, appropriateness, and affordability are key components of this vision.

Essential medicines, especially new formulations, are often not available to the poorest people in the world because these medicines are too expensive. Much of the activity around the 'access to essential medicines' has focused on this point and possible solutions proposed such as increasing generic competition and voluntary discounts on branded medicines. Global procurement and local production have also been proposed as sustainable ways of building robust supply chains that enhance availability and accessibility.

The last part of the 'access to essential medicines' vision focuses on appropriateness, that is, rational prescribing practices and use of essential medicines. This point is relevant to all settings. However, it is also vital that essential medicines are suitable for a specific purpose, context and environment. Formulations that are heat stable, can be given orally rather than intravenously, and can be given in appropriate dose sizes, particularly for essential paediatric medicines, have obvious advantages for low-income settings.

Because of the lack of market forces to conduct research and development (R&D) into treatments for diseases that only affect poor people, such as the tropical diseases human African Trypanosomiasis (sleeping sickness) and Chagas disease, this vital area has been neglected until recently. International campaigns and the work of WHO's Intergovernmental Working Group on Public Health, Innovation and Intellectual Property *(38)* have helped to focus on the specific issues involved in the R&D for the treatment of most neglected diseases and explore some possible solutions, such as increasing PPPs and alternative incentives for research in this area. Such activities help to make essential medicines increasingly available, accessible, appropriate, and affordable.

2.4.2 Access to appropriate medical devices

Given that the key components involved in the agenda to improve access to appropriate medical devices are availability, accessibility, appropriateness, and affordability, it is easy to see the similarities with

Box 2.3 The differences in medical devices and pharmaceuticals

Medical devices differ from pharmaceuticals in various ways.

Diversity
Medical devices vary in size, complexity, packaging, and use.

Innovation
Innovation of medical devices results primarily from clinicians' insights, rather than laboratory exploration. Medical devices undergo incremental improvements, with a relatively short commercial life-cycle of about 18 months on average *(39)*.

Durability
Medical devices have a wide range of durability with extremes ranging from a few minutes for disposable devices, to several decades for some implantable devices and medical equipment.

Mode of action
Medical devices, as such, do not achieve their principal intended action in or on the human body by pharmacological, immunological, or metabolic means, although some (e.g. syringes) may be used to deliver medicines.

Medical devices produce mainly local and physical effects on the body rather than systemic and pharmacological effects.

Regulation
The extent of regulatory scrutiny of medical devices is based on the risk class attached to their use.

Assessment of safety and efficacy for low-risk classes of medical devices can be performed by the manufacturer. For high-risk classes of medical devices, bibliographic evidence may be submitted to the competent authorities to prove safety and efficacy *(40)*.

Efficacy or effectiveness of medical devices is proven before they are put on the market. However, clinical effectiveness (i.e. when a device produces the effect intended by the manufacturer relative to the medical conditions) is more difficult to prove.

Supply
About 80% of the medical device industry is made up of small and medium enterprises.

Distribution of heavy medical equipment is usually costly.

There is no well-defined supply chain or profession (such as pharmacists for pharmaceuticals) involved in the supply of medical devices.

Usage
The performance of a device depends not only on the device itself but also on how it is used.

The user interface of a medical device is usually not direct (device–patient) except for assistive devices, but in many cases involves an intermediary (device–operator–patient).

There is often a learning curve associated with the use of medical devices, particularly for complex high-tech devices, with a need for technical training and support.

Medical devices may require service and maintenance.

Many medical devices are used for diagnostic purposes.

Many medical devices are used to alleviate functional disabilities (most commonly referred to as assistive products).

Sources: *(39, 41, 42)*

the 'access to essential medicines' agenda. However, before simply replacing the term "medicines" with "medical devices", it is important to stress how medical devices differ from medicines. Box 2.3 outlines those key differences, and the factors listed show that if the agenda to improve access to appropriate medical devices has any chance of being successful, some specific issues should be carefully considered. Merely following in the footsteps and practices of the 'access to essential medicines' is not enough. The agenda to improve access to medical devices requires, and deserves, its own unique agenda.

The following chapters in this section discuss in some detail the areas of the medical device landscape—supply, regulation, and innovation—that need to be considered in order to understand the concepts behind the agenda to improve access to appropriate medical devices.

2.5 The medical device market

"The medical device industry is one of the most vital and dynamic sectors of the economy" *(43)*. Revenue from sales of medical devices worldwide was estimated at a little over US$ 210 billion for 2008 *(39)*. This is double the estimated revenue for 2001, giving an annual growth rate of about 6%. These sales figures are being achieved by an industry that comprises more than 27 000 medical device companies worldwide and employs altogether about one million people *(39)*.[6]

Four fifths of global medical device sales revenue comes from sales in the Americas and Europe *(44)* (Figure 2.1). Ten countries account for nearly 80% of world sales revenue, with the United States at the top of the list (41%), followed by Japan (10%),

---

6   For more information on medical devices companies worldwide, see AdvaMed (http://www.advamed.org), MEDEC (http://www.medec.org), Medical Technology Association of Australia (http://www.mtaa.org.au) and AusBiotech (http://www.ausbiotech.org) (accessed 17 July 2010).

Figure 2.1 Medical device markets by region (% sales revenue), 2009*

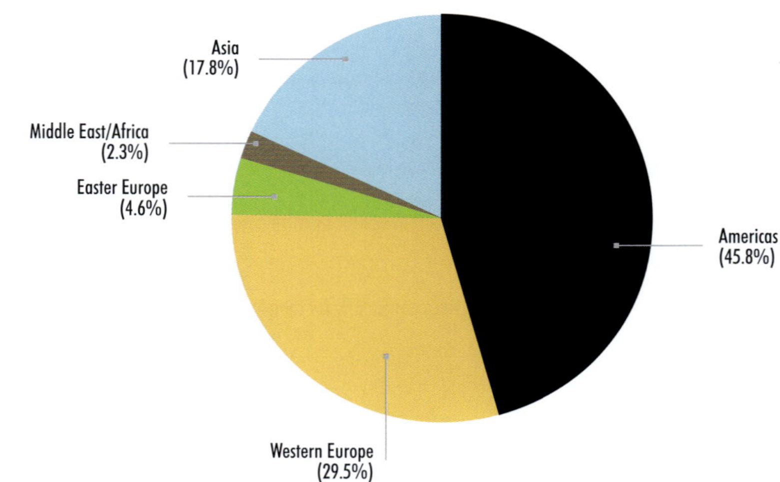

*Based on **The world medical markets fact book 2009 (44)**, which provides estimates based on the 67 countries for which sufficient data are available and which account for more than 90% of total medical device sales revenue.

Germany (8%), and France (4%) *(44)* (Table 2.1). Figure 2.2 shows the breakdown of the market by type of medical device.

Table 2.2 lists the top 30 medical device companies by sales revenue *(45–74)*. All but 11 have their headquarters in the United States. Together, these 30 companies account for 89% of the estimated US$ 210 billion in global sales revenue. Since there are about 27 000 medical device companies in the world, the remaining 11% of global sales revenue must be shared by a vast number of manufacturers in the small and medium enterprise (SME) category.

Historically, virtually all high-tech medical devices have been made by manufacturers in, or based in, industrialized countries. Low-tech devices, such as

Table 2.1 Top ten countries by sales revenue, 2009*

		Sales revenue US$ (millions)	%
1	United States	91 316	40.7
2	Japan	22 721	10.1
3	Germany	18 147	8.1
4	France	8 625	3.8
5	Italy	8 004	3.6
6	United Kingdom	7 628	3.4
7	China	6 161	2.7
8	Spain	4 887	2.2
9	Canada	4 757	2.1
10	Switzerland	4 063	1.8
Subtotal		176 309	78.6
World total (67 countries)		224 103	100

*Based on The world medical markets fact book 2009 *(44)*, which provides estimates based on the 67 countries for which sufficient data are available and which account for more than 90% of total medical device sales revenue.

Figure 2.2 World medical markets by sector (% sales revenue), 2009*

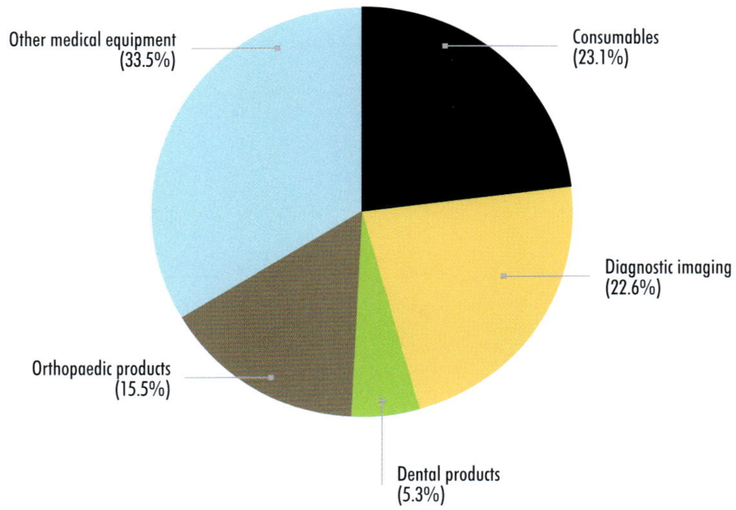

*Based on **The world medical markets fact book 2009 (44),** which provides estimates based on the 67 countries for which sufficient data are available and which account for more than 90% of total medical device sales revenue.

Table 2.2 Top 30 medical device companies by sales revenue, 2008*

	Company	Headquarters	Sales revenue US$ (millions)
1	Johnson & Johnson	United States	23 225
2	GE Healthcare	United States	17 392
3	Siemens Healthcare	Germany	15 526
4	Medtronic	United States	13 515
5	Baxter International	United States	12 400
6	Covidien	Ireland	9910
7	Philips Healthcare	Netherlands	9227
8	Boston Scientific	United States	8050
9	Becton Dickinson	United States	7156
10	Stryker	United States	6718
11	B. Braun	Germany	5263
12	Cardinal Health	Ireland	4600
13	St. Jude Medical	United States	4363
14	3M Health Care	United States	4293
15	Zimmer	United States	4121
16	Olympus	Japan	3920
17	Smith & Nephew	United Kingdom	3801
18	Hospira	United States	3620
19	Terumo	Japan	3400
20	Danaher Corporation	United States	3227
21	Synthes	United States	3206
22	Beckman Coulter	United States	3099
23	Alcon	Switzerland	2881
24	Fresenius Medical Care	Germany	2875
25	C.R. Bard	United States	2452
26	Abbott	United States	2241
27	Dentsply	United States	2194
28	Varian Medical	United States	2070
29	Biomet	United States	2135
30	Dräger	Germany	1729
			185 734

*Data derived from company annual reports (45–74). Not all data refer strictly to medical devices: for those companies that compete in several industrial sectors, most do not differentiate between sales revenues from medical devices and those from other products.

Table 2.3 Sales revenue from medical devices in middle-income countries, 2009*

		Sales revenue US$ (millions)	%
1	China	6161	28.6
2	Brazil	2606	12.1
3	Mexico	1890	8.8
4	India	1617	7.5
5	Turkey	1062	4.9
6	Malaysia	826	3.8
7	South Africa	701	3.2
8	Thailand	661	3.1
9	Colombia	530	2.5
10	Iran	465	2.2
11	Argentina	419	1.9
12	Egypt	416	1.9
13	Venezuela	371	1.7
14	Romania	355	1.6
15	Cuba	345	1.6
16	Chile	309	1.4
17	Viet Nam	288	1.3
18	Croatia	255	1.2
19	Belarus	253	1.2
20	Ukraine	249	1.1
21	Bulgaria	229	1.1
22	Lithuania	201	0.9
23	Serbia	199	0.9
24	Indonesia	194	0.9
25	Pakistan	184	0.8
26	Peru	183	0.8
27	Philippines	163	0.8
28	Morocco	152	0.7
29	Jordan	144	0.7
30	Latvia	141	0.6
Subtotal		21 569	100
World total (67 countries)		224 103	100

*Based on *The world medical markets fact book 2009 (44)*, which provides estimates based on the 67 countries for which sufficient data are available and which account for more than 90% of total medical device sales revenue.

condoms, surgical gloves, simple dressings, gauze, syringes, and hypodermic needles have been manufactured in emerging economies (e.g. India, Indonesia, Malaysia, and Sri Lanka, among others). Moreover, most of the multinational companies listed in Table 2.2 have established manufacturing sites in developing countries. Table 2.3 shows 30 middle-income countries that are producing medical devices: their total sales account for an estimated 10% of the world market. The top five countries by projected sales revenue—China, Brazil, Mexico, India, and Turkey—account for 60% of the total middle-income country market (and 6% of the world market).

2.6 Medical device regulation

By definition, a regulatory system is a set of rules. For manufactured products, such as medicines, vaccines and medical devices, the rules serve to limit the risk of a product causing harm (being unsafe) or not fulfilling its intended purpose (being ineffective) or not complying with standards of quality (being substandard).

In general, a government body is responsible for drawing up the rules, for enacting them into national law and for ensuring that the law is enforced. Those required to comply with the rules are those who make the products (manufacturers), who sell them (vendors) and who use them (users). The users of medical devices are in most cases health professionals (nurses, physicians, surgeons, etc.), who are usually subject to regulatory oversight by the respective professional bodies to which they belong. Box 2.4 gives an historical overview of regulation.

Several components make up the "regulatory framework" that is common to the countries manufacturing the vast majority of medical devices in use today—Australia, Canada, Japan, the United States, and the European Union countries. These components comprise, at a minimum *(81)*:

- the regulatory rules;
- a government-approved regulatory authority (to enforce the rules);
- one or more "conformity assessment bodies" (which are accredited by a European Union Member State and may issue market approval) to assess whether a manufacturer or a device conforms to regulatory requirements;
- a classification scheme that ranks devices by level of potential risk associated with their use (three or four levels, or "classes", are generally used, with most devices in the low and moderate risk classes, and less than 10% in the moderate-to-high risk class);
- a quality assurance or management system, managed by the manufacturer, to ensure compliance of a device with quality standards and norms;
- a system for evaluating the clinical safety and performance of a device;
- a system for granting marketing (market entrance) approval for a device that complies with the regulatory rules; and
- a surveillance system capable of detecting and investigating adverse events associated with the actual use of a device on the market.

Box 2.4 An historical overview of medical device regulation

Historically, countries have tended to introduce regulation or tighten existing regulation only when forced to do so by public outcry over an unexpected dramatic event. Food was the first object of regulatory concern. A scare in the United States over adulterated foods precipitated the creation, in 1906, of the FDA, the world's first national regulatory authority *(75)*. By the mid-1930s medicines had moved into the public limelight: in 1937, the deaths of over 100 Americans who had taken a cough mixture containing an antifreeze-type chemical caused the FDA to add pre-market testing to their medicinal regulatory requirements *(76)*. Then, in the 1960s, came an international outcry over thalidomide, a sedative responsible for congenital defects in more than 10 000 babies in 46 countries: the outcry jolted many regulatory authorities, particularly in Europe, to tighten their oversight.

Regulation, however, came relatively late to the medical device world. A major public concern in the 1960s and 1970s was the risk of micro-shock from an electrical current via devices connected to patients *(41)*. During the 1970s and 1980s, demand for stronger regulatory legislation arose from serious adverse effects caused by intrauterine contraceptive devices (the Dalkon shield and the Copper-7 device) and several brands of tampons *(77)*.

Beginning in the 1970s, Australia, Canada, the European Union countries, Japan and the United States, which together account for close to 85% of the device market share, led the way in strengthening their regulatory systems *(78)*. In 1976, the United States Government overhauled its regulatory framework for "food, drugs and cosmetics" (which also covered medical devices) and continued to refine and strengthen it with additional amendments, with the latest ones in 2007 *(79)*.

In Europe, too, the regulatory environment became more stringent, although mainly to enhance the cohesion of a single internal European market. Beginning in 1990, the European Union (EU) introduced in all its Member States an approach to medical device regulation based on mandatory "essential requirements" of safety, performance, and quality. This approach had the overall aims of "ensuring the functioning of the internal market and a high level of protection of human health and safety" *(80)*.

By mid-2009, 76 of WHO's Member States had some form of regulatory capacity (see Table 2.4).

Table 2.4 Countries with a system for regulating medical devices

Albania	Hungary	Paraguay
Argentina	Iceland	Peru
Australia	India	Philippines
Austria	Indonesia	Poland
Bahrain	Ireland	Portugal
Belgium	Italy	Republic of Korea
Bolivia	Iraq	Romania
Brazil	Japan	Russian Federation
Bulgaria	Kazakhstan	Saudi Arabia
Canada	Kenya	Serbia
Chile	Kuwait	Singapore
China	Latvia	Slovakia
Colombia	Liechtenstein	Slovenia
Costa Rica	Lithuania	South Africa
Croatia	Luxembourg	Spain
Cuba	Malaysia	Sweden
Cyprus	Malta	Switzerland
Czech Republic	Mexico	Thailand
Denmark	Malta	Turkey
Ecuador	Mexico	Ukraine
Egypt	Netherlands	United Arab Emirates
Estonia	New Zealand	United Kingdom
Finland	Nicaragua	United States of America
France	Norway	Uruguay
Germany	Pakistan	Venezuela
Greece	Panama	Viet Nam

*irrespective of how complete (or incomplete) the regulatory system.
Sources: *(82–86)*.

2.7 An introduction to medical device innovation

Medical device innovation refers not only to the invention of new devices but also to adjustments to, or incremental improvements of, existing devices and clinical practices. It also denotes efforts to adapt devices designed for use in one setting, such as a modern high-tech hospital, to be used in another setting, such as a patient's home. WHO defines innovation as a "process cycle of three major phases that feed into each other: discovery, development and delivery" *(38)*. Public health need creates a demand for products of a particular kind, suited for the particular medical, practical, or social context of a group, and feeds into efforts to develop new or improved products.

Innovation of medical devices must demonstrate added value for patient health. Yet, even when clear benefits exist, the technology may be rejected simply because it is new, threatens existing practices, or has costs that outweigh benefits *(87)*.

Technological development in health care differs from technological development in other fields. Among other things, in the health-care context, technological development may be influenced by the emotional factors attached to health and illness as well as by a broad political commitment to provide people with the latest medical technologies *(88)*.

However, innovation can bring much more than technological benefits. The promise of innovation attracts research grants for hospitals, laboratories, and physicians' practices. Patient groups, health planners, health economists, government officials, regulators, managers, and health-care insurers together form a complex aggregation of sometimes contradictory forces whose interplay determines the pattern of innovation uptake. Together, these forces constitute important factors of demand for new medical technologies. They also influence how the technologies will be used, integrated into mainstream care, and distributed, financed, evaluated, and monitored. In many cases, physicians may tip the balance in favour of or against the acceptance of a new medical device *(87)*.

The supply side—medical device manufacturers—also have a substantial role to play. The vitality of the medical device industry is reflected in its focus on R&D and innovation. Many medical devices undergo constant "incremental" development based on feedback from users and on advances in technology, thereby producing keen competition among manufacturers.

Traditionally, though, it has been the smaller companies that are most active and innovative in R&D *(87)*. According to a research consultancy commissioned by the FDA in 2006, in the United States small companies play a greater role in R&D of new medical devices, with large firms providing organizational and capital assets that help ensure the commercial success of new products *(89)*. The barriers to medical device innovation and possible solutions to overcome them are discussed in detail in Section 5.

2.7.1 Applying non-medical innovation to health care

Many medical devices initially emerged not from clinical research but from technologies developed in other areas. This phenomenon is referred to as "dual use"

Dual use technologies include lasers, ultrasound, MRI, spectroscopy, and information technology. MRI, for example—a non-invasive technology used to diagnose injury to body organs from trauma, tumours and infarction—grew out of basic research on the structure of atoms. Other examples of technologies incorporated into health care that came from outside the medical research field include Internet communication, shock wave technology (now used in lithotripsy), and devices devised by the army for use in difficult field conditions, which can often serve as a model for the design of medical devices to be used in remote low-resource settings *(91)*.

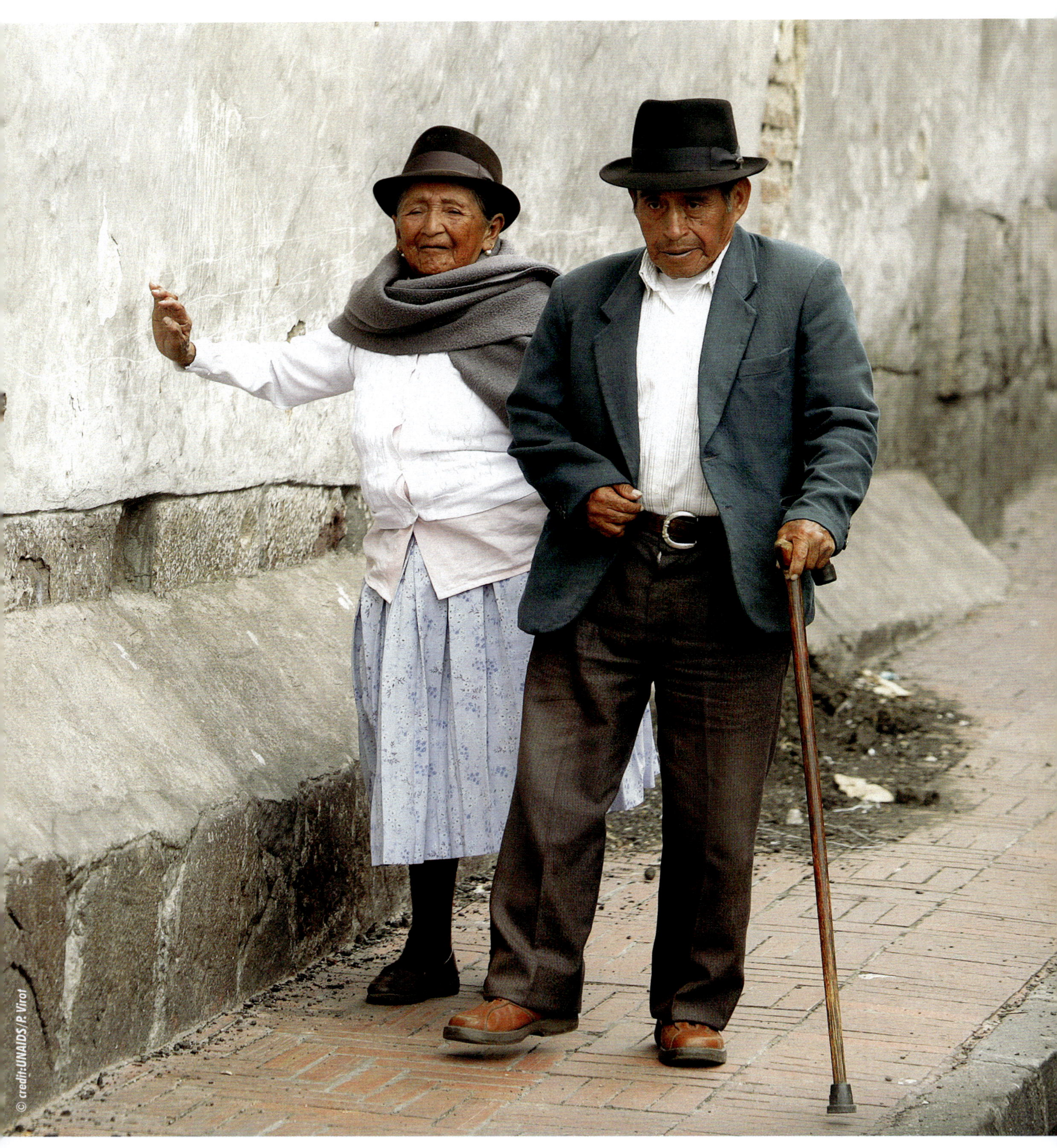
© credit:UNAIDS/P. Virot

Public health needs

Public health priorities are defined by the diseases and risk factors that cause the highest morbidity and mortality, and the disabilities that cause the greatest functional impairment. Identifying the high-burden medical conditions, diseases, disabilities and risk factors is an important step in developing global public health needs assessments and subsequent research agendas. However, the local context is also important. In order to bring maximum benefit to their populations, individual countries should also address the health needs of their citizens by using robust national public health needs assessments to build their national health plans and develop their research plans. Countries may also find the national or regional case-mix configuration (the type or mix of patients treated by a hospital or specific region) useful in devising their public health needs assessments and national health plan.

Research in medical devices is needed for the diseases and disabilities that account for most of the illnesses, deaths and functional difficulties that currently affect people worldwide. Historically, developing countries have a higher burden of communicable diseases than from noncommunicable diseases. However, some developing countries are emerging more quickly than others from this traditional disease pattern and have begun to be affected by noncommunicable diseases, such as diabetes, cancer, and cardiovascular diseases, which used to dominate only industrialized countries.

Research needs and priorities of high-resource countries differ in many respects from those of low-resource countries, and at present, nearly all medical device research is conducted in high-resource countries, being focused on the needs of these countries.

Unfortunately, public health needs are currently not the main driver of medical device research. Manufacturers often research and develop devices for diseases that will net the most profit. The crucial components of the agenda to improve access to appropriate medical devices—availability, accessibility, appropriateness, and affordability—are strikingly absent. The necessary health-based stepwise approach to choosing medical devices is discussed below.

3

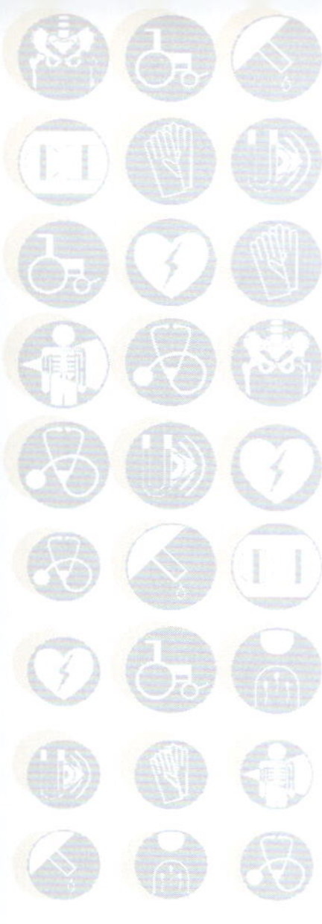

3.1 A health-based approach to choosing medical devices

Medical devices are used for a wide range of purposes and health problems. They are often chosen largely for their technical or technological attributes. And often, the choice is influenced by considerations not directly related to health, such as persuasive marketing, commercial image-building and physician preferences.

A major objective of the *PMD* project was to develop an approach to choosing medical devices that is based, first and foremost, on the need for a positive health outcome. The proposed approach takes as its starting point a simple question: What medical devices are needed to meet public health problems? It then seeks to answer a less simple question: among devices that are available, which could fulfil that need? The project proposes a stepwise approach, which is discussed in Box 3.1.

3.2 Identifying current and future public health needs

Preventive, diagnostic and therapeutic medical devices have a direct relationship to the diagnosis of a specific disease and can be prioritized according to burden of disease. Specific units of measurement can be used by researchers to indicate the magnitude and impact of disease burden and disability. Such indicators can be used as a guide to deciding which diseases and disabilities should be priority targets of future research. Commonly used indicators include disability-adjusted life years (DALYs), years lived with a disability (YLD) and the percentage of total disease burden due to major risks to health. These indicators, while not perfect—particularly for areas of the world where robust data on disease, death and, disability are lacking—can be used to deduce public health needs and to compare the potential cost-effectiveness of different interventions in reducing disease burden (1). They can therefore also be used as guides for resource allocation (93).

Table 3.1 lists the 15 diseases that contribute most to the global burden of disease as measured by DALYs estimated for 2004, DALY projections for 2030, and YLD for 2004.

Future projections of high-burden diseases show an increase in noncommunicable and chronic conditions, such as cardiovascular diseases, chronic obstructive pulmonary disease, diabetes, and hearing loss, and a decrease in the burden caused

Box 3.1 The stepwise approach to meeting public health problems

The first step in this approach is to identify the most important health problems. For a regional health policy-maker or national government official, disease burden estimates, such as WHO's global burden of disease analyses, may be useful. Countries can match this type of evidence with their health goals. For a hospital manager, the most commonly encountered diseases reported among the hospital's catchment population or case load could also help define priority targets. This initial step aims to seek information about the diseases or disabilities that are the highest priority in terms of public health needs, select evidence-based clinical guidelines for managing the diseases, identify care pathways and protocols, and evaluate the available resources. Global disease burden or disease risk factor estimates may again provide the needed information. For individual countries, public health needs assessments conducted as part of the national health plan are also necessary. In addition, the case-mix configuration (the type or mix of patients treated by a hospital) nationally and/or regionally might be of use.

The second step in this approach is to identify how health problems are best managed. Clinical guidelines are an obvious source of information for clinical decision-making. Guidelines do, however, give limited information on which devices should be used for a given procedure. Standard care pathways and protocols can contribute in identifying which medical devices are needed in the management of a disease.

The third step is to link the results of the first two steps and produce a list of medical devices needed for the management of the identified high-burden diseases, at a specific health-care level and in a given context. This step involves identifying the category of devices and then the specific models of devices required to perform the required procedures (92). To complete this step requires knowledge about the intended purpose, design, safety, effectiveness, durability, and technical specifications of the many devices in the local context.

A STEPWISE APPROACH TO IDENTIFY MEDICAL DEVICES FOR PUBLIC HEALTH NEEDS

A consistent and comparative description of the burden of diseases and injuries and the risk factors that cause them is an important input to health decision-making and planning processes. The WHO global burden of disease (GBD) measures burden of disease using the disability-adjusted life year (DALY). This time-based measure combines years of life lost due to premature mortality and years of life lost due to time lived in states of less than full health.

Countries can match this type of evidence with their health goals and policies, epidemiologic status and resources to decide how to set their health agenda.

Identify disease burden of the target population

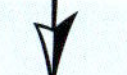

Select the associated evidence-based clinical guidelines

Identify care pathways and protocols

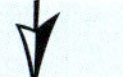

List medical devices according to the protocols
Distinction is to be made between preventive, diagnostic, therapeutic and assistive medical devices

Matrix of the medical devices needed in the management of the identified diseases

Use a horizontal approach to identify existing resources.

Evaluate the gap between the matrix and the available resources.

Apply a medical devices management system.

A STEPWISE APPROACH TO IDENTIFY ASSISTIVE MEDICAL DEVICES FOR PUBLIC HEALTH NEEDS

Identify disease burden of the target population

Link disease to level of functioning through the International Classification of Functioning, Disability and Health (ICF) core sets

International Classification of Functioning, Disability and Health (ICF) describes relevant problems in the functioning of patients with specific diseases or health problems.
www.icf-research-branch.org.

Map ICF core set to assistive products according ISO 9999 classes using document N19 rev

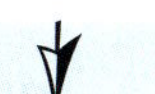

An ICF coreset is a selection of ICF classes representing relevant aspects in the functioning of the people with a specific disease or health problem.

ISO 9999:2007 establishes a classification of assistive products especially produced, or generally available, for persons with disability.

http://www.iso.org/iso/iso_catalogue/

The N19 rev is a product of ISO/TC173/SC2/WG11; in this document a linkage is made between divisions of ISO 9999 with relevant ICF-classes.

The document is available on www.rivm.nl/who-fic

List of assistive products (classified according to ISO 9999) for the management of the disability (functioning problems) associated to each disease burden of the target population

Table 3.1 Estimated disability-adjusted life years (DALYs) and years lived with disability (YLD)[a] for 15 leading causes of disease burden worldwide, 2004 and 2030

Estimated DALYs,[b] 2004	% total	Projected DALYs, 2030 (baseline scenario)	% total	Estimated YLD,[c] 2004	% total
Perinatal conditions[d]	8.3	Unipolar depressive disorders	6.2	Unipolar depressive disorders	10.9
Lower respiratory infections	6.2	Perinatal conditions[d]	5.6	Hearing loss, adult onset	4.6
Diarrhoeal diseases	4.8	Ischaemic heart disease	5.5	Refractive errors (not cataracts)	4.6
Unipolar depressive disorders	4.3	Road traffic accidents	4.9	Maternal conditions	3.9
Ischaemic heart disease	4.1	Cerebrovascular disease	4.3	Alcohol use disorders	3.7
HIV/AIDS	3.8	Chronic obstructive pulmonary disease	3.8	Perinatal conditions[d]	3.4
Cerebrovascular disease	3.1	Lower respiratory infections	3.2	Cataracts	3.0
Road traffic accidents	2.7	Hearing loss, adult onset	2.9	Osteoarthritis	2.6
Tuberculosis	2.2	Refractive errors[e]	2.7	Chronic obstructive pulmonary disease	1.9
Malaria	2.2	HIV/AIDS	2.5	Road traffic accidents	1.7
Chronic obstructive pulmonary disease	2.0	Diabetes mellitus	2.3	Alzheimer and other dementias	1.6
Refractive errors[e]	1.8	Malignant neoplasms (lung and stomach)	2.2	Diabetes mellitus	1.6
Hearing loss, adult onset	1.8	Cataracts	1.9	Ischaemic heart disease	1.4
Alcohol use disorders	1.6	Alcohol use disorders	1.9	Cerebrovascular disease	1.2
Diabetes mellitus	1.3	Diarrhoeal diseases	1.6	Diarrhoeal diseases	1.0

a   DALY, disability-adjusted life year; YLD, years lived with a disability.
b   Standard DALYs by cause (3% discounting, age weights).
c   Standard YLD by cause (3% discounting, age weights).
d   Causes arising in the perinatal period as defined by the International Classification of Diseases; does not include all conditions occurring in the perinatal period.
e   Prevalence estimates for low vision and blindness due to specific disease and injury, revised to take into account the WHO analysis of regional distributions for causes of blindness. A recent WHO analysis of surveys that measured presenting vision loss was used to estimate YLD for an additional cause — "refractive errors". Previous global burden of disease estimates for vision loss based on "best corrected" vision did not include correctable refractive errors.
Source: *(95).*

Table 3.2 DALYs for selected risk factors and high-burden diseases

Risk factor	% of total DALYs	Outcomes (corresponding to selected high-burden diseases)
Childhood underweight	5.9	Diarrhoeal diseases, malaria, perinatal conditions from maternal underweight
Unsafe sex	4.6	HIV/AIDS
Alcohol use	4.5	Ischaemic heart disease, stroke, diabetes, malignant neoplasms, depression
Unsafe water, sanitation and hygiene	4.2	Diarrhoeal diseases
High blood pressure	3.7	Diabetes, ischaemic heart disease, cerebrovascular disease
Tobacco use	3.7	Malignant neoplasms, chronic obstructive pulmonary disease, tuberculosis, diabetes, vascular disease
Suboptimal breastfeeding	2.9	Diarrhoeal diseases, lower respiratory infection
High blood glucose	2.7	Diabetes, ischaemic heart disease, cerebrovascular disease
Indoor smoke from solid fuels	2.7	Lower respiratory disease, lung cancer, chronic obstructive pulmonary disease
Overweight and obesity	2.3	Ischaemic heart disease, stroke, diabetes

Source: *(95).*

by communicable diseases, such as diarrhoeal diseases, tuberculosis, and malaria *(94)*. Table 3.2 lists the risk factors that contribute to high-burden diseases, calculated as a percentage of total DALYs for all causes.

3.2.1 Disability

More than 600 million people worldwide currently live with disabilities *(96)*, 80% of which live in developing countries; most are poor and have limited or no access to basic services, including rehabilitation facilities. The causes of disability include chronic disease, injury, violence, infectious disease, malnutrition and conditions associated with poverty. But what is meant by the term "disability"?

After centuries of debate, there is now general consensus about what constitutes a disability as recently shown by the implementation of the International Classification of Functioning, Disability and Health *(97)* and the UN Convention on the Rights of Persons with Disabilities *(98)*. Both the ICF and the Convention view disability as the outcome of complex interactions between health conditions and features of an individual's physical, social, and attitudinal environment that hinder his or her full and effective participation in society.

The ICF classifies functioning and disability, and is used to describe problems in human functioning. It complements the International Statistical Classification of Diseases and Related Health Problems (ICD-10) *(99)*, which contains information on diagnosis and health condition, but not on functional status.

The ICF contains over 1450 classes of functioning aspects. An ICF core set is a selection of ICF classes representing relevant aspects in the functioning of people with a specific disease or health problem *(97)*. Currently, there is no "bridge" to help identify the assistive products needed by persons with disabilities resulting from the selection of high-burden diseases as described above. This report attempts to provide such a bridge *(32)*.

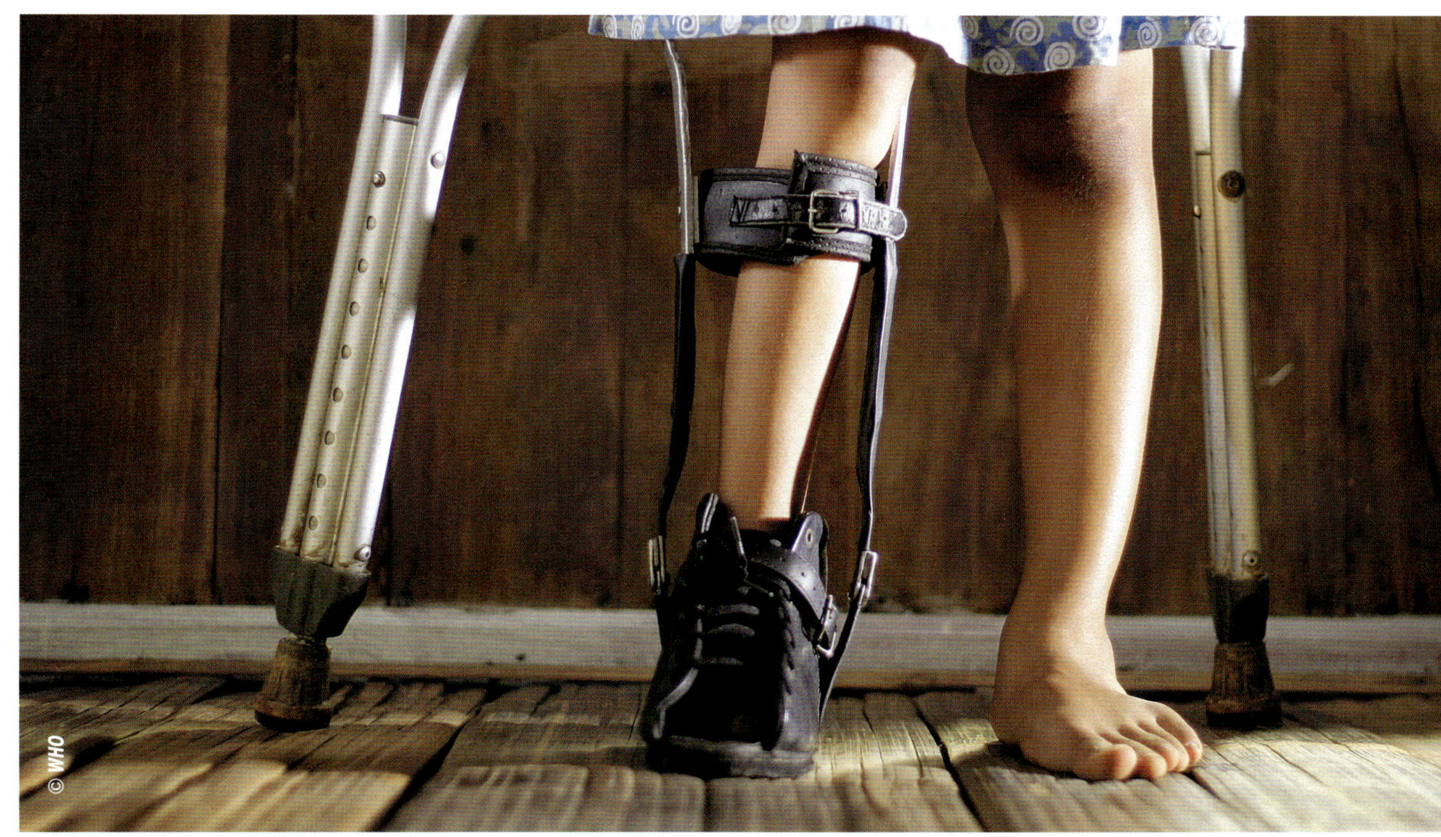

3.2.2 Global trends

Targeting research on medical devices for the management of disease or disability must, increasingly, take into account regional trends and differences in the proportional burden of these diseases and disabilities.

Globally, life expectancy is increasing, with more and more people living well into their 80s and 90s *(100)*. Variations in life expectancy still exist within the less developed regions *(101)*. Ageing populations, however, are growing more quickly in less developed than in developed countries. Although older populations in Asia and Africa still live predominantly in rural areas, this situation is likely to reverse over the next 20–30 years due to the growing urbanization of ageing populations *(102, 103)*. Living longer is associated with co-morbidity (the presence of several illnesses at the same time) and with chronic debilitating conditions, such as coronary heart disease, diabetes, cancer, dementia, and osteoarthritis.

The ageing of populations, coupled with decreasing fertility and birth rates, is projected, for some countries, to lower population size, reduce the labour force, increase old-age dependency and generally raise the average frequency of ill-health and disability *(104)*. These trends, in turn, are set to raise demand for medical devices needed in old age, such as labour-saving technologies; for devices adapted to home care and telemedicine; and for the training of patients and caregivers on using medical devices at home.

In addition to the growing incidence of noncommunicable diseases, developing countries are affected by diseases of poverty. These include communicable diseases, maternal ill-health, perinatal and nutrition-related conditions, malaria, and other parasitic diseases. Together, they account for over half the burden of disease in these countries—ten times the burden of these same diseases in industrialized countries *(94)*. In addition, while traffic-related deaths and injuries occur in virtually all regions, their incidence in developing countries is twice that in industrialized countries, and is growing *(105)*.

Figure 3.1 shows commonalities and disparities in disease patterns between different WHO regions. All regions show a downward trend for communicable diseases. Tuberculosis, lower respiratory infections, diarrhoeal diseases, HIV/AIDS, malaria, and perinatal conditions are all expected to decline across WHO regions in the next two decades, with the exception of HIV/AIDS, which is expected to increase slightly in the European Region, to become a chronic condition.

The projected disparities between WHO regions concern mainly noncommunicable, chronic conditions, and road traffic accidents. COPD, road traffic accidents, ischaemic heart disease, lung and stomach cancer, and cerebrovascular disease are expected to fall in the European Region and in the Region of the Americas but to rise in the Eastern Mediterranean, South-East Asia, and Western Pacific Regions. Diabetes is increasing across all regions, with the Americas likely to experience a greater increase over time than other regions. In the African Region, most chronic conditions are increasing, with the exception of ischaemic heart disease and depression, which are declining. Road traffic accidents are projected to rise considerably in the African and South-East Asia Regions.

Urbanization

In 2008, 3.3 billion people—more than half of the human population—were living in cities or towns. Urban growth rates are highest in developing countries, which absorb an average of 5 million new urban residents every month and account for 95% of the growth of the world's urban population *(103)*. Urbanization is expected to increase dramatically in certain areas, notably the largely rural areas of Asia and Africa.

By 2050, the urban population of developing countries will reach 5.3 billion, with Asia expected to host 63% (3.3 billion people) and Africa nearly 20% of the world's urban population (1.3 billion people). By contrast, the urban population of industrialized countries is expected to remain largely unchanged, rising slightly from just over 900 million in 2005 to 1.1 billion in 2050. Low natural growth in the population and declining fertility rates contribute to this trend *(106)*.

The majority of urban residents will be poor, while at the same time access to health care in cities will become increasingly difficult. In the world's megacities, the burden of disease is shifting towards

Figure 3.1 Changing disease patterns across WHO Regions, 2004 and 2030[a]

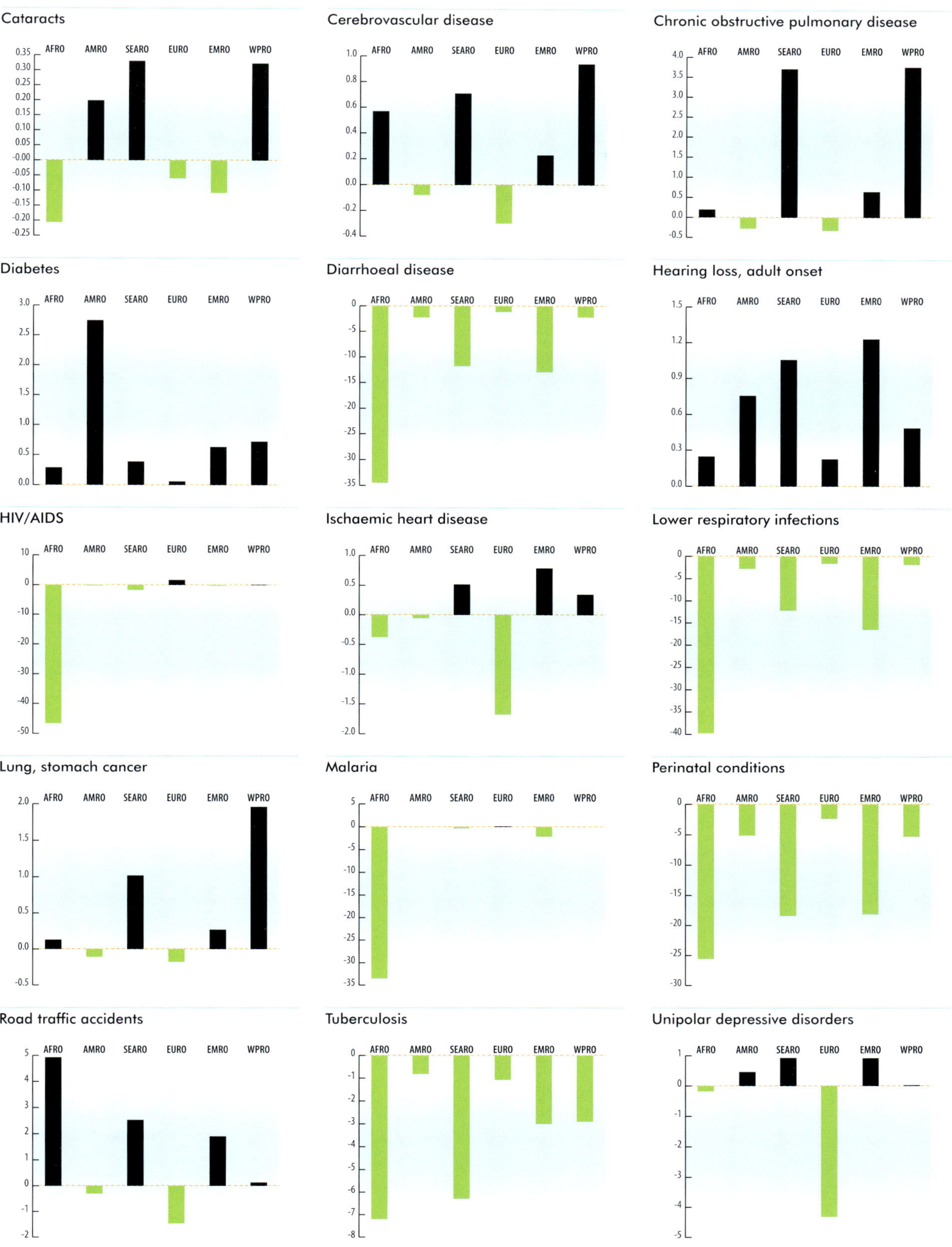

a   For each high-burden disease the sum of the DALY (Disability-adjusted life year). burden over the entire age distribution for 2004 was divided by the total population. This was repeated for 2030. To calculate the change in DALY burden the $\sum$(DALY burden per capita (2004) − DALY burden per capita (2030)) for each of the WHO regions was performed.

AFRO, WHO African Region; AMRO, WHO Region of the Americas; SEARO, WHO South-East Asia Region; EURO, WHO European Region; EMRO, WHO Eastern Mediterranean Region; WPRO, WHO Western Pacific Region.

A positive value (black) reflects an increase in the per capita DALY burden over time. A negative value (green) reflects a decrease in the per capita DALY burden over time. The scale of the Y axis for the different diseases varies as the numbers vary in function of the disease and whether the change in time is large or small. For example, a small difference implies either that the condition did not have a high burden in the area or that there is little change over time.

Source: **(24).**

noncommunicable diseases. Road traffic will increase air pollution and the frequency of injuries. Spreading slum areas will increase the incidence of diarrhoeal diseases.

Growing urban populations together with population ageing are expected to heighten the need for primary health care including appropriate medical devices *(107)*.

Health workers in short supply

The health workforce is a key building block of any health system and a priority target of strategies to strengthen health systems *(108)*. Currently there is a worldwide shortage of more than 4 million doctors, nurses, midwives and other health workers, according to WHO estimates *(109)*. The shortage is most critically felt in sub-Saharan Africa but also in South-East Asia, where the needs for health professionals are immense, particularly in Bangladesh, India, and Indonesia. There is a global need for more trained health professionals. Research, too, needs to explore ways of replacing the workforce by technology— particularly technology for diagnosis, monitoring and health-care delivery in remote settings or where trained staff are not present in sufficient numbers. Moreover, the need for labour-saving technology is expected to intensify with falling birth and fertility rates, rising life expectancy, and a growing chronic disease burden *(104)*.

To be of any value in coming years, research agendas that link public health needs to appropriate innovations in medical devices must take these trends into account.

3.3 Public health: the missing research target

Research related to medical devices is driven largely by the need for better solutions and for greater technological capabilities, and also by promising ideas, scientific interest and economic considerations. Research related to medical devices is mainly targeted to high-resource countries, which effectively fails to adequately address global public health needs. The discrepancy in health research funding (the "10/90 gap"), is one contributing factor

to the research discrepancy. The main drivers of medical device research are also contributing factors.

3.3.1 Drivers of research

The forces driving medical device research come from three main sectors: academia, industry, and public research foundations

Academia

The drive to improve public health and medical devices is powerful among many scientists, physicians, and biomedical engineers; so, too, is their interest in discovering new theories and solutions that advance scientific knowledge. Much research takes place in university, medical or engineering faculties. Research strategies at academic institutions are typically driven by professors' research interests and by the compatibility of a proposed research project with prevailing academic opinions. They are also influenced by the ability to acquire research grants and therefore by the priorities of funding bodies. Individual researchers or research teams, including scientists, clinicians and engineers, normally submit their ideas for peer review. The reviewers base their assessment on the scientific and/or engineering credibility of the ideas, their originality, and the extent to which they are innovative.

Traditionally, academic research receives most of its funding from governments, research foundations and commercial entities, each exerting a specific influence on research protocols and research objectives. Research proposals funded by public research programmes, such as the National Institutes of Health in the United States and European research councils, focus primarily on basic research, originality and the robustness of the proposed methodology. Translating ideas into products for manufacture has typically been outside the funding remit of the councils. Public funding for translational research, however, is on the increase, at least in some countries, notably the United Kingdom.

Scientists are also motivated by the prospect of achieving recognition among their peers by publishing their work in peer-reviewed journals and thereby enhancing their careers and the likelihood of receiving further research grants, a prospect that is also attractive to host universities. By attracting outstanding scientists, a university raises its academic status.

Historically, managing the transfer of knowledge from academia to industry has been difficult, given the differences in timetables, expectations, outcomes and working culture, as well as the resulting difficulties of communication and collaboration between the two sectors *(110)*.

Industry

Although there are numerous economic, social and political factors that influence research and innovation, medical devices are developed largely through a bottom-up approach whereby manufacturers explore with health professionals and other device users ideas for developing new, or for improving existing, products. Much of this work is achieved through an iterative process or through adaptation of existing technologies.

The area of research interest funded by commercial sources rarely goes beyond the market focus of the funder, so that the researcher may be less free to explore or to respond to emerging evidence, or to satisfy his or her curiosity *(110)*. Moreover, research funded by industry is generally "applied" to specific industry targets, although it often builds on the more basic academic research.

Large manufacturers have their own funds for research, whereas smaller firms like academic spin-off companies depend on external sources of capital, especially venture capital and capital provided by public policy initiatives *(111)*. Even so, large firms are finding it increasingly difficult to maintain their R&D spending levels. Some even resort to purchasing intangibles (such as know-how or innovative ideas), at relatively moderate cost, from university researchers and start-up firms with the appropriate technology—a practice that is not limited to the medical device arena.

The medical device industry invests in R&D for three main reasons: 1) the likelihood of substantial returns on R&D investment; 2) the status of R&D as a core element of a company's business model; and 3) a perceived need to strengthen and expand the presence of the company in markets, including

emerging markets *(45–74)*. In this regard, ready access to capital is a strong facilitating factor *(111)*. Table 3.3 shows the ratio of investment to R&D of some manufacturers.

An additional driver of industry R&D is progress being made in enabling technologies by researchers in disciplines not directly related to medical devices: materials science, semiconductor technology, batteries, memory chips, energy management, and computer capabilities, to name a few examples.

Industry's research needs differ between mature and emerging markets. Emerging medical device markets, such as India, the Russian Federation, and Turkey, are catching up with mature markets, such as Australia and the United States. However, emerging markets are at a disadvantage due to the lack of appropriate infrastructure, trained staff and logistics, and of an established system to accommodate the introduction of new solutions.

The major medical device manufacturers spend an average of 7.5% of their sales revenue on R&D (Table 3.3). Annual company reports for 2008 describe the marketing strategy of industry in mature and emerging markets in general terms rather than defining specific research agendas targeting public health needs.

The main drivers of industry research on medical devices intended for emerging markets are the growing commercial appeal of these markets and the opinions of health-care professionals trained in the use of medical devices by industry *(45–74)*. Leading manufacturers of medical devices see an opportunity for increasing their sales revenue in the emerging markets of developing economies. *(45, 46, 48, 50, 57, 61, 63, 66–70)*.

In certain countries affected by HIV/AIDS and tuberculosis, some companies set their market goals and their support strategies, such as training and direct cash donations, to coincide with government initiatives for improving laboratory systems and services *(51)*.

Some leading companies base their research strategies on the need to maintain their market lead,

Table 3.3 Industry R&D investment by ratio of R&D to sales revenue, 2008[a]

	Manufacturer	Headquarters	Revenue from sales US$ (millions)	R&D investment US$ (millions)	% ratio R&D sales
1	Boston Scientific	United States	8050	1006	12.5
2	St. Jude Medical	United States	4363	532	12.3
3	Siemens Healthcare	Germany	15 526	1630	10.5
4	Philips Healthcare	Netherlands	9227	892	9.7
5	Medtronic	United States	13 515	1275	9.4
6	Beckman Coulter	United States	3099	280	9.0
7	C.R. Bard	United States	2452	199	8.1
8	Johnson & Johnson	United States	23 225	1858	8.0
9	Dräger	Germany	1729	136	7.8
10	Olympus	Japan	3920	289	7.4
11	Alcon	Switzerland	2881	204	7.1
12	Baxter International	United States	12 400	868	7.0
13	Varian Medical	United States	2070	136	6.5
14	Hospira	United States	3620	214	6.0
15	Danaher Corporation	United States	3227	190	5.9
16	Becton Dickinson	United States	7156	396	5.5
17	Stryker	United States	6718	368	5.5
18	Synthes	United States	3206	170	5.3
19	Terumo	Japan	3400	175	5.2
20	Zimmer	United States	4121	194	4.7
21	Smith & Nephew	United Kingdom	3801	152	4.0
22	B. Braun	Germany	5263	181	3.4
23	Covidien	Ireland	9910	340	3.4
24	Fresenius Medical Care	Germany	2874	80	2.8
25	Dentsply	United States	2194	52	2.4
			157 947	11 817	7.5

a   Data derived from company annual reports (45–74). Not all data refer strictly to medical devices: for those companies that compete in several industrial sectors, most do not differentiate between sales revenues from medical devices and those from other products. Not all companies report R&D expenditure specifically for medical devices.

on demographic trends and/or on the rising demand for cutting-edge medical technology in emerging economies (47, 59, 60).

Governments and public research foundations

Governments and public institutions have an incentive to invest in basic research and specifically in biomedical technology because of the proven benefit to public health of such research (111).

The German Research Foundation (DFG), for example, funds research in basic science, which promotes innovation at universities and other publicly financed institutions. Projects supported by the DFG cover research on medical devices that have scientific merit rather than on the magnitude of the public health burden that the devices resulting from the research might help to reduce. The foundation is thus free to fund a research proposal concerning, say, genetic tests for the diagnosis of rare diseases. A senior DFG medical adviser notes that such a decision, however, would not be taken as part of a routine policy but rather on the grounds of a personal scientific interest (112). This method of selecting research topics runs the risk of disregarding public health needs.

The European Commission urges its high-income Member States to spend about 3% of their gross domestic product on the development of cutting-edge technologies to promote innovation, without specifying public health issues *(113)*. Without explicit reference to public health needs, however, the political and economic motivation to invest in advanced technology can turn the attention of public health officials away from public health priorities to a supposed need for highly sophisticated devices. The outcome may be an increased competitive advantage for individual countries but at the same time a disregard for technology that could have a strong global impact on public health *(114)*.

However, in October 2009 the European Commission initiated an exploratory process on the future of the medical devices sector to overview existing public health and industrial challenges, to identify current dynamics of the sector and to highlight key topics of interest at the European level. The list of issues identified by a wide range of stakeholders were: (1) future challenges and opportunities for public health and medical technologies developments; (2) balance between the patients' needs and financial sustainability; and (3) competitiveness and innovation of the medical devices industry *(115)*.

3.4 The gap

In the preparation of this report, no research agendas specifically developed for medical devices—or even mentioning medical devices—could be found through searches in documents produced by institutions concerned with health research, such as the World Bank, the Organisation for Economic Co-operation and Development (OECD), the International Monetary Fund (IMF), and the Global Forum for Health Research. Published reports on research often group medical devices together with precision instruments or laboratory equipment, which are not strictly medical devices. Data on research expenditures specifically for medical devices are often incomplete or absent. One exception was The European Commission's Directorate-General

for Research, which is working on a structured research agenda that spans all European Union countries and that links research on medical devices to priority health needs within the scope of the European Union's Seventh Framework Programme for Research and Technological Development *(6, 116)*. This programme has a budget of €6 billion for the period 2007–2013. Within the programme, the European Commission's Community Research and Development Information Service (CORDIS)[1] defines three broad areas of activity for small- and medium-sized high-tech, research-intensive enterprises:

1. biotechnology, generic tools and technologies for human health;
2. translating research for human health; and
3. optimizing the delivery of health care.

CORDIS highlights additional research topics, including neurological diseases, infectious diseases, cancer, cardiovascular diseases, diabetes and obesity, rare diseases, other chronic diseases, as well as all technological areas related to health biotechnologies, biomedical engineering, medical technologies and bioinformatics *(116)*.

Conspicuously absent is any comprehensive consideration of the crucial components of the agenda to improve access to appropriate medical devices—availability, accessibility, appropriateness, and affordability—to help formulate possible future research agendas that encourage development of medical devices to meet the priority public health needs of developing countries.

Therefore, the aim of the fact-finding research components of this report (described in Section 4) was to identify key information and knowledge gaps necessary to form the basis of a possible research agenda. A suggested research agenda to better align public health needs with medical device research, which considers the crucial components of availability, accessibility, appropriateness, and affordability, is discussed in Section 6.

---

1   http://cordis.europa.eu/fp7/health/home_en.html (accessed 17 July 2010).

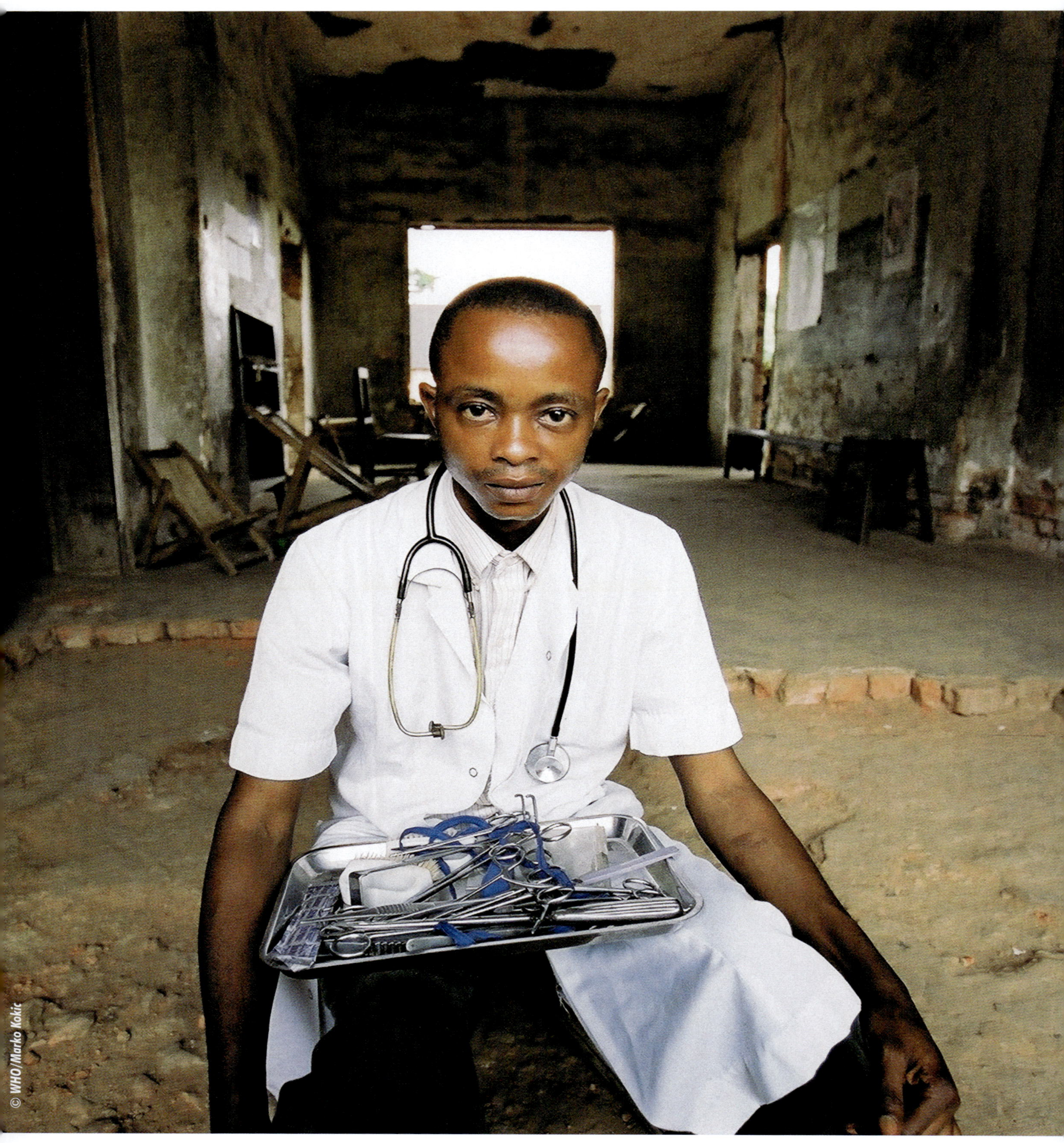

Priority Medical Devices project: methods used

As mentioned in Section 1, the two objectives of this report are to 1) inform national health policy-makers, international organizations, manufacturers and other stakeholders (including users of medical devices) of the factors preventing the current medical device arena from achieving its full public health potential; and 2) to provide a basis on which all players in the medical device scene can, together, use the findings of this report to help make public health the central focus of their activities. This can be most effectively done by proposing a research agenda for appropriate medical devices that adequately addresses public health needs.

In order to fulfil these objectives, it was necessary to conduct some fact-finding research, develop a methodology to identify the gaps between access to medical devices and clinical need, and identify the barriers and possible solutions to improve global access to appropriate medical devices. This research was overseen by the Advisory Group of the *PMD* project and facilitated by informal consultations. A Steering Group helped to oversee the writing of this report.

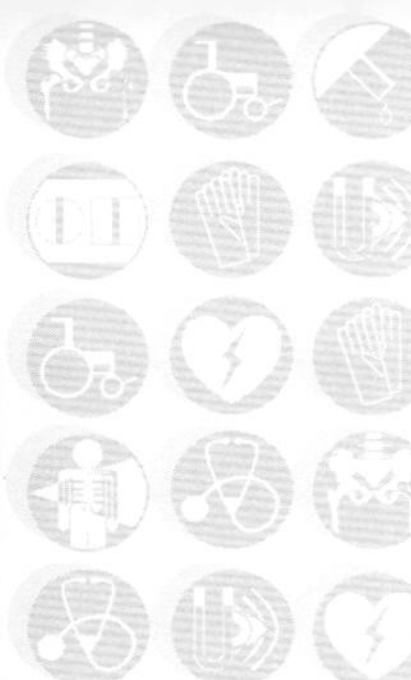

4.1 Methodology

4.1.1 Identifying key medical devices in high-burden diseases

The starting point was to map the high-burden diseases according to the *Global Burden of Disease (GBD) and Risk Factors (1)*—an entity that was discussed in detail in Section 3. Following this mapping exercise, relevant evidence-based clinical guidelines, developed to describe the management of 15 high-burden diseases, were selected to identify the medical devices recommended for the management of a specific disease in clinical practice *(92)*. Only clinical guidelines published after 2000 were included and selected separately for all 15 high-burden diseases and disabilities where the title referred to the disease or disability. At the start of the project in 2007, WHO had developed guidelines for eight of the selected 15 high-burden diseases.

Clinical guidelines rarely provide a table containing all medical devices needed in the treatment of a particular disease. In some cases, the clinical procedure was mentioned in general terms (e.g. oral examination) without mentioning the specific medical devices used in this procedure. In such cases, the exam name is listed in the matrix followed by "equipment" (e.g. oral examination equipment).

For the purpose of the *PMD* project, medical devices were extracted from the clinical guidelines by two independent reviewers. Each reviewer independently scored the guidelines. Where interpretations differed, a specialist in the specific disease area was consulted who had the final word.

All medical devices (or techniques that involve medical devices) identified in the selected clinical guidelines were included in an "Availability Matrix" that formed the baseline of medical devices needed to manage the disease. Medical devices were categorized as preventive, diagnostic, therapeutic and assistive devices, according to the stages of health care. For these four subcategories, a distinction was made between medical devices for general use (e.g. stethoscope or thermometer) and disease-specific medical devices *(92)*.

4.1.2 Identifying the medical device gap

Few data exist on the availability and use of medical devices to treat disease and assist people with functioning. Most countries do not have a centralized database showing medical device use. Therefore, in order to identify gaps in the use of the key medical devices for the 15 global high-burden diseases, it was necessary to develop specific methodologies. Two pilot surveys were devised and validated, one for countries and one for specialists, to gather quantitative and qualitative information about medical device gaps *(92)*. In addition, specialist focus groups, round-table discussions and individual consultations helped to provide valuable qualitative information.

Six countries were selected according to Human Development Index (HDI) level—A, B, C, D, E and F. The questionnaire included questions around medical devices for three representative high-burden diseases: diabetes mellitus—an example of a noncommunicable disease; tuberculosis (TB) —an example of infectious disease; and road traffic accidents—an example of a condition for which early intervention could prevent long-term disability. Common points between each disease questionnaire included the following: distinguishing between diagnostic, therapeutic, and assistive devices; questions on medical devices for general (non-disease specific) use (e.g. hospital beds); the appropriate use of medical devices, that is, questions about the management and availability of technical information, communication materials, and training opportunities of medical devices during various stages of the device's life-cycle (e.g. at time of procurement and daily use); and questions about the future local or regional needs that respondents felt were important. The questionnaire was sent to in-country WHO representatives who then forwarded the survey to the respective Ministry of Health and key health care-related associations in each selected country.

This country survey was adapted to form a specialist questionnaire that contained medical device-related questions on each of 15 high-burden diseases. This questionnaire was sent directly to appropriate specialists in each of the high-burden diseases. The specialist survey was designed to help identify any clinical problems associated with the medical devices recommended for each high-burden medical condition. The selected specialists were also encouraged to suggest clinical areas that may require further medical device research.

These specifically designed and validated questionnaires, combined with a comprehensive literature search and review, were used as the basis for identifying the evidence for, and experience of, medical device innovation, choosing and using medical devices, and identification of the problems and challenges in these key areas, as well as possible ways of overcoming these barriers. Medical device activities were categorized in this way (i.e. medical device innovation and choosing and using medical devices) because these categories cover the processes and stages involved in the agenda to improve access to appropriate medical devices, and are directly or indirectly associated with the crucial 4 components—availability, accessibility, appropriateness, and affordability.

For a detailed description of all of the methodologies used in the fact-finding research in this report *(92)*.

4.2 Results

4.2.1 Identifying key medical devices in high-burden diseases

Table 4.1 shows the clinical guidelines selected for each of the 15 global high-burden diseases and disabilities.

Table 4.1 Selected clinical guidelines for 15 high-burden diseases

GBD code	GBD cause/ sequelae	Source guideline	Guideline title	Publication year	Settings
U003	Tuberculosis	WHO	Treatment of tuberculosis: guidelines for national programmes	2003	Primary, secondary and tertiary care, low/ medium resource
U009	HIV/AIDS	WHO	Antiretroviral therapy for HIV infection in adults and adolescents: recommendations for a public health approach	2006	Primary, secondary and tertiary care, low/ medium (/high) resource
U010	Diarrhoeal diseases	USAID, UNICEF, WHO	Diarrhoeal treatment guidelines for clinic-based healthcare workers	2005	Clinic and home, low resource
U020	Malaria	WHO	Guidelines for the treatment of malaria	2006	Primary care, low/ medium resource
U039	Lower respiratory infections	Scottish Intercollegiate Guidelines Network	Community management of lower respiratory tract infections in adults, a national clinical guideline	2002	Primary care, high resource
U049,U050, U051, U052	Perinatal conditions: Low birth weight, birth asphyxia and birth trauma, other perinatal conditions	WHO	Managing newborn problems: a guide for doctors, nurses and midwives	2003	Inside and outside hospital, low (/medium) resource
U067	Malignant neoplasms	Scottish Intercollegiate Guidelines Network	Management of patients with lung cancer: a national clinical guideline	2005	Primary, secondary and tertiary care, high resource
		Scottish Intercollegiate Guidelines Network	Management of oesophageal and gastric cancer: a national clinical guideline	2006	Primary, secondary and tertiary care, high resource
U079	Diabetes mellitus	WHO	Guidelines for the prevention, management and care of diabetes mellitus	2006	Primary, secondary and tertiary care, low/medium/high resource
U082	Unipolar depressive disorders	National Institute for Health and Clinical Excellence	Depression: management of depression in primary and secondary care	2007	Primary and secondary care, high resource
U100	Cataracts	Philippine Academy of Ophthalmology	Clinical practice guideline for the management of cataract among adults	2001, updated 2005	Primary, secondary and tertiary care, medium resource
U102	Hearing loss, adult onset	WHO	Primary ear and hearing care training resource, advanced level	2006	Primary care, low resource
U107	Ischaemic heart disease[i]	Veterans Health Administration, Department of Defense, USA	VA/DoD clinical practice guideline for the management of ischaemic heart disease	2003	Primary and secondary care, high resource
U108	Cerebrovascular disease	Stroke Foundation New Zealand	Life after stroke: New Zealand guideline for management of stroke, best practice evidence-based guideline	2003	Primary, secondary and tertiary care, high resource
U112	Chronic obstructive pulmonary disease	National Collaboration Centre for Chronic Conditions	National clinical guideline on management of chronic obstructive pulmonary disease in adults in primary and secondary care	2004	Primary and secondary care, high resource
U150	Road traffic accidents	WHO	Guidelines for essential trauma care	2004	Hospital, low/medium/high resource

Source: *(92).*

Table 4.2. Availability Matrix: example of tuberculosis

GBD code	GBD cause	Case definition	Clinical Procedure	Medical device							
				Preventive		Diagnostic		Therapeutic		Assistive	
				General	Specific	General	Specific	General	Specific	General	Specific
U003	Tuberculosis	Cases refer to individuals with clinical tuberculosis, normally pulmonary sputum culture positives and extra-pulmonary cases	Management of HIV sero-negative/positive cases (pulmonary TB)			X-ray, microscope and laboratory equipment	Equipment to obtain diagnostic specimens, culture test and facilities, sputum smear test, tuberculin test	Surgical equipment (late complications)			
			Management of extrapulmonary TB								

Source: **Treatment of tuberculosis: guidelines for national programmes.** Geneva, World Health Organization, 2003.

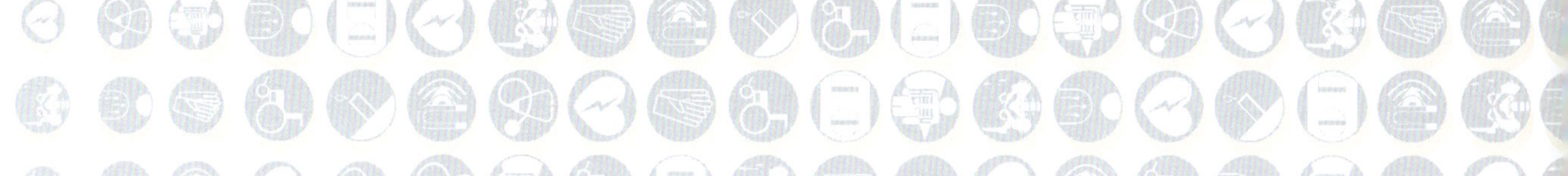

Table 4.3 Availability Matrix: example of diabetes mellitus

GBD code	GBD cause	Case definition	Clinical Procedure	Medical device								
				Preventive		Diagnostic		Therapeutic		Assistive		
				General	Specific	General	Specific	General	Specific	General	Specific	
U079	Diabetes Mellitus	Cases of DM	Management of venous plasma concentration of 11.1 mmol/L 2 h after a 75 g oral glucose challenge	Tape measure, weighing scale, blood pressure meter, diagnostic tests on metabolic syndrome, screening tests for diabetic dyslipidaemia	—	Tape measure, weighing scale, blood pressure meter, cardiovascular examination devices, equipment for chemistry panel, fasting lipid profile test, urinalysis equipment, thyroid stimulating hormone test, ECG	OGTT, blood glucose measuring test, urine glucose measuring test, HBA1c measuring test, autoimmune marker tests (HLA type, ICA, anti-GAD)		HBA1c measuring test, whole blood and plasma glucose measuring equipment (FPG), self-monitoring blood glucose device		—	
		Atherosclerosis	Management of atherosclerosis due to diabetes			Screening tests for risk factors for macrovascular disease						
		Diabetic Foot and Amputation	Management of chronic or recurring diabetic foot ulcers, Surgical elimination of the lower extremity or part of it			Tuning fork, monofilament, Doppler ultrasonography, arteriography		Angioplasty, surgical instruments		Specially fitted shoes, plantar support		
		Neuropathy	Management of reflexes and vibration loss; damage and dysfunction of sensory, motor, or autonomic nerves			Reflex hammer, tuning fork, monofilament						
		Retinopathy-blindness	Management of microaneurysms or eye blood vessel damage and Management of blindness			Ophthalmoscope (coupled with biomicroscope), visual acuity test, non-mydriatic camera		Laser and surgical equipment				
		Nephropathy	Management of renal failure due to diabetes			Urinary microalbumin test, serum creatinine test, serum lipids test, creatinine clearance test		Dialysis equipment, kidney transplantation equipment				

Anti-GAD, antibodies to glutamic acid decarboxylase; DM, Diabetes Mellitus; ECG, electrocardiogram; FPG, fasting plasma glucose test; HLA, human leukocyte antigen; ICA, islet-cell cytoplasmic antibodies; OGTT, oral glucose tolerance test.
Source: *Guidelines for the prevention, management and care of diabetes mellitus.* Geneva, World Health Organization, 2006.

Table 4.4 Availability Matrix: example of road traffic accidents

GBD code	GBD cause	Case definition	Clinical Procedure	Medical device							
				Preventive		Diagnostic		Therapeutic		Assistive	
				General	Specific	General	Specific	General	Specific	General	Specific
U150	Road traffic accidents	Includes crashes and pedestrian injuries due to motor vehicles	Airway management	—	—	Laryngoscope, fibre-optic endoscope, transilluminator, equipment for capnography	Oesophageal detector device (bulb, syringe or electric)	Tongue depressor, suction device, suction catheter, suction tubing, stiff suction tip, bag-valve-mask, Magill forceps	Basic trauma pack Equipment to perform basic oral/nasal airway management, endotracheal tube with tube connector, needle/surgical cricothyroidotom		
			Management of respiratory distress			Stethoscope, pulse oximeter	Arterial blood gas measurements	Oxygen supply equipment, face mask with tubing, nebulization mask, venture mask, needle and syringe, chest tubes, bag-valve-mask or mechanical ventilator	Basic trauma pack, nasal cannulae and prongs, underwater seal drainage bottle, needle and tube thoracotomy		
			Management of shock			Clock, stethoscope, blood pressure cuff, electronic cardiac monitor, laboratory facilities for measurement of electrolytes, arterial blood gasses, haematocrit, haemoglobin, creatinine, glucose, lactate, thermometer, weighing scale, fluid warmers	Central venous pressure monitor, pulmonary capillary wedge pressure monitor	Gauze and bandages, intravenous infusion set, equipment for central venous infusion (central lines), urinary catheter, nasogastric tube, equipment to perform splinting, equipment for blood transfusion	Arterial tourniquet, intraosseous needle and lines, right-heart catheterization, deep interfascial packing		
			Management of head injury			Torch, CT scan	Intracranial pressure monitoring	Operating theatre equipment, surgical equipment (to perform craniotomy, craniectomy, treatment of intracerebral haematoma), ventilator, equipment for nasogastric feeding	Equipment to maintain cerebral perfusion and oxygenation, cerebrospinal fluid drains		
			Management of neck injury			Contrast radiography, endoscope, angiography		Operating theatre equipment, surgical equipment	Packing, balloon catheter tamponade		
			Management of chest injury			Stethoscope, pulse oximeter	Arterial blood gas measurements	Operating theatre equipment, chest tubes, oxygen supply equipment, equipment to perform anaesthesia, equipment for rib and intrapleural block	(Pulmonary) Thoracotomy equipment, prosthetic graft, pulmonary resection equipment		
			Management of abdominal injury			Blood pressure cuff, stethoscope, ultrasound, CT scan	Diagnostic peritoneal lavage equipment, abdominal tap equipment	Operating theatre equipment	Laparotomy equipment		
			Management of extremity injury			X-ray, image intensification equipment		Surgical equipment, implants, amputation equipment, equipment to perform splinting, splint, sling	External fixation equipment (pins and plaster), equipment for irrigation and debridement of wounds, fasciotomy	Immobilization device, wrapping device, fixation device	Spine board
			Management of spinal injury			X-ray, CT scan, MRI scan		Surgical equipment	Cervical spine traction device	Immobilization devices (spine board)	Cervical spine brace (halo device)
			Management of burns and wounds					Sterile dressing material, surgical equipment	Dermatome, equipment to perform escharotomy, skin grafting, splinting, reconstructive surgery		Splints
			Rehabilitation			Electromyograph					Splints, prostheses

CT, computerized tomography; MRI, magnetic resonance imaging.
Source: **Guidelines for essential trauma care.** Geneva, World Health Organization, 2004.

These selected clinical guidelines were used as the basis for extracting key medical devices recommended for the 15 global high-burden diseases and disabilities. All extracted medical devices were logged in an "Availability Matrix." Tables 4.2–4.4 illustrate the Availability Matrix for three of the 15 diseases and disabilities—tuberculosis, diabetes, and road traffic accidents. (Please see *(92)* for the complete Availability Matrix).

4.2.2 Identifying the medical device gaps

Results from four countries

Four of the six countries responded to the country survey. Countries A and B, responded via the Internet. Countries D and C, responded via hard copy. Responses from country D, consisted of 22 questionnaires, one having been filled out completely, and the others having been completed partially by 21 different officials. Responses from countries A, B and C, were received as a single response. To be able to report on the countries consistently, the 22 responses of country D were amalgamated into one. Please see *(92)* for the quantitative results of the questionnaire which illustrate the percentage of clinical procedures for TB, diabetes, and road traffic accidents. Results are shown by country and health-care level, disease, and the percentage "yes"

answers on the use of diagnostic, therapeutic, and assistive medical devices for the three conditions surveyed.

In all four countries, almost all devices for each condition surveyed are reported as being used in the tertiary health-care level. The primary health-care level shows the fewest numbers of devices in use, while the secondary health-care level shows more devices are employed. The use of diagnostic and therapeutic devices for TB in the four countries differs. All devices are reported to be in use at the tertiary health-care level, while those at the primary and secondary levels show that use is only slightly less frequent.

The reported use of assistive devices for TB shows a similar pattern of use as for road traffic accidents. Assistive devices are in use at the tertiary health-care level in all countries, but for the other health-care levels, only two countries use them.

For diabetes, all four countries are consistent in reporting assistive devices in use at the tertiary level. Country C is the only country reporting a large percentage of assistive devices at all health-care levels.

Table 4.5 Priority conditions and medical devices identified by countries

Disease[a]	Country A	Country B	Country C	Country D
Disease 1	**Airway disease (Asthma)**	**Diabetes**	**Acute heart failure**	**Diabetes**
Medical devices associated	X-ray machines, pulse oximeters, nebulizers, inhalers	Blood pressure machine; glucometers, stethoscopes, diagnostic sets	Promotion and prevention, medical assistance[b]	Insulin pump
Disease 2	**Ischaemic heart disease**	**TB**	**Cancer**	**Cancer**
Medical devices associated	electrocardiogram (ECG) machines, lab equipment for angiography/angioplasty	X-ray, laboratory microscope, laboratory incubator, water bath, centrifuge, X-ray film-processor	Promotion and prevention, medical assistance[b]	Diagnostic equipment
Disease 3	**Road traffic accidents**	**Injuries**	**Cardiovascular disease**	**Cardiovascular disease**
Medical devices associated	X-ray imaging devices, orthopaedic equipment, medical supplies for resuscitation	C-arm X-ray machine, diathermy machine, suction machines, orthopaedic instruments, orthopaedic operating table, anaesthetic machines, theatre operating lamp, patient ventilators, ECG monitors, infusion pumps	Promotion and prevention, medical assistance[b]	Pacemaker, defibrillator

a   Disease 1 indicates highest priority; Disease 2, second-highest priority; Disease 3, third-highest priority.
b   These activities are not medical devices.

Countries B and D, do not indicate any difficulty with regards to access to technical information. Country A, reports difficulties accessing technical information on procurement, maintenance and use of medical devices in relation to the three conditions. Only country C reports a lack of access to technical information on maintenance/repair and daily use of medical devices for diabetes.

For medical devices in general use, the gaps are smaller: only country A, reported that accessibility of technical information associated with maintenance and repair of devices is lacking for diabetes and road traffic injuries.

Table 4.5 shows each country response in identifying the three most pressing diseases or disabilities (and the associated medical devices needed in their management) emerging over the next five years. These conditions are listed in descending order. The majority of the diseases indicated are noncommunicable diseases. Medical devices indicated by the respondents are mainly diagnostic and therapeutic devices.

Results of the specialist surveys

Response rate to the specialist survey was 35%. Forty-six per cent of the respondents were from low-income settings, 30% from middle-income settings, and 24% from high-income levels. The specialist survey found that low-income settings have a dearth of technical information—for procurement, maintenance and repair, and daily use. Gaps between need and availability of devices are greatest in low-income settings. A lack of assistive devices was also indicated (except for wheelchairs and crutches).

4.3 Identifying key assistive products for high-burden diseases

Assistive products to help functionality problems associated with 15 high-burden diseases and disabilities need special attention. The initial research conducted for the purposes of this report highlighted the scale to which access to appropriate assistive products has been neglected to date (outlined below). Furthermore, the fact that assistive devices were not mentioned in any of the priority needs in the country surveys further underscores this point.

Currently, no global burden of disability has been developed. Moreover, most clinical guidelines do not mention assistive products. In fact, the clinical guideline identified very few, if any, assistive products required to help functioning for those with the 15 high-burden diseases and disabilities. Therefore, to assess the assistive product gap, a different concept had to be used. The *PMD* project attempted to develop a linking methodological process that would help to identify assistive products needed by people with disabilities resulting from the selection of high-burden diseases. This process was complex and included a five step approach: 1) identification of 15 high-burden diseases by using the GBD; 2) description of ICD-10 and ICF as complementary systems; 3) bridging the GBD and ICF through core sets and functioning profiles; 4) delineating the ISO 9999; and 5) relating the ICF to the ISO 9999. The full methodology of this approach is described in detail in *(32)*.

As a result, the project was able to bridge the 15 high-burden diseases to functions through ICF core sets. For those diseases where a core set did not exist, a functioning profile was developed and the results are shown in Table 4.6. (In order to follow the rationale of this process and to better understand Table 4.6, see *(32))*.

This methodological process has helped with the first step of the health-based approach to choosing assistive products (i.e. indentifying need). However, much more research is required to give assistive products and functioning disabilities the same time, attention, effort, and resources given to medical devices and diseases.

Table 4.6 Selected high-burden diseases and their associated core sets or functioning profiles

GBD code	GBD cause/sequela	ICF core set available for the disease		No ICF core set available for the disease	
		ICF core set for the general disease	ICF core set available for one or more forms of the disease	Functioning profile based on expert opinions	Functioning profile based on guidelines and literature
U003	Tuberculosis	No	No	Yes	No
U009	HIV/AIDS	No	No	Yes	No
U010	Diarrhoeal diseases	No	No	No	Yes
U020	Malaria	No	No	Yes	Yes
U039	Lower respiratory infections	No	No	No	Yes
U050, U051, U052	Low birth weight, birth asphyxia and birth trauma, other perinatal conditions	No	No	Yes	No
U067	Malignant neoplasms	No	Yes, for breast cancer, and head and neck cancer	No	Yes, for colon cancer and lung cancer
U079	Diabetes mellitus	Yes	No	No	No
U082	Unipolar depressive disorders	Yes, for depression	No	No	No
U100	Cataracts	No	No	No	Yes
U102	Hearing loss, adult onset	No	No	No	Yes
U107	Ischaemic heart disease	Yes	No	No	No
U108	Cerebrovascular disease	Yes, for stroke	No	No	No
U112	Chronic obstructive pulmonary disease	Yes	No	No	No
U150	Road traffic accidents	No	No	Yes, for lower extremity, and upper extremity	No

Source: *(32)*

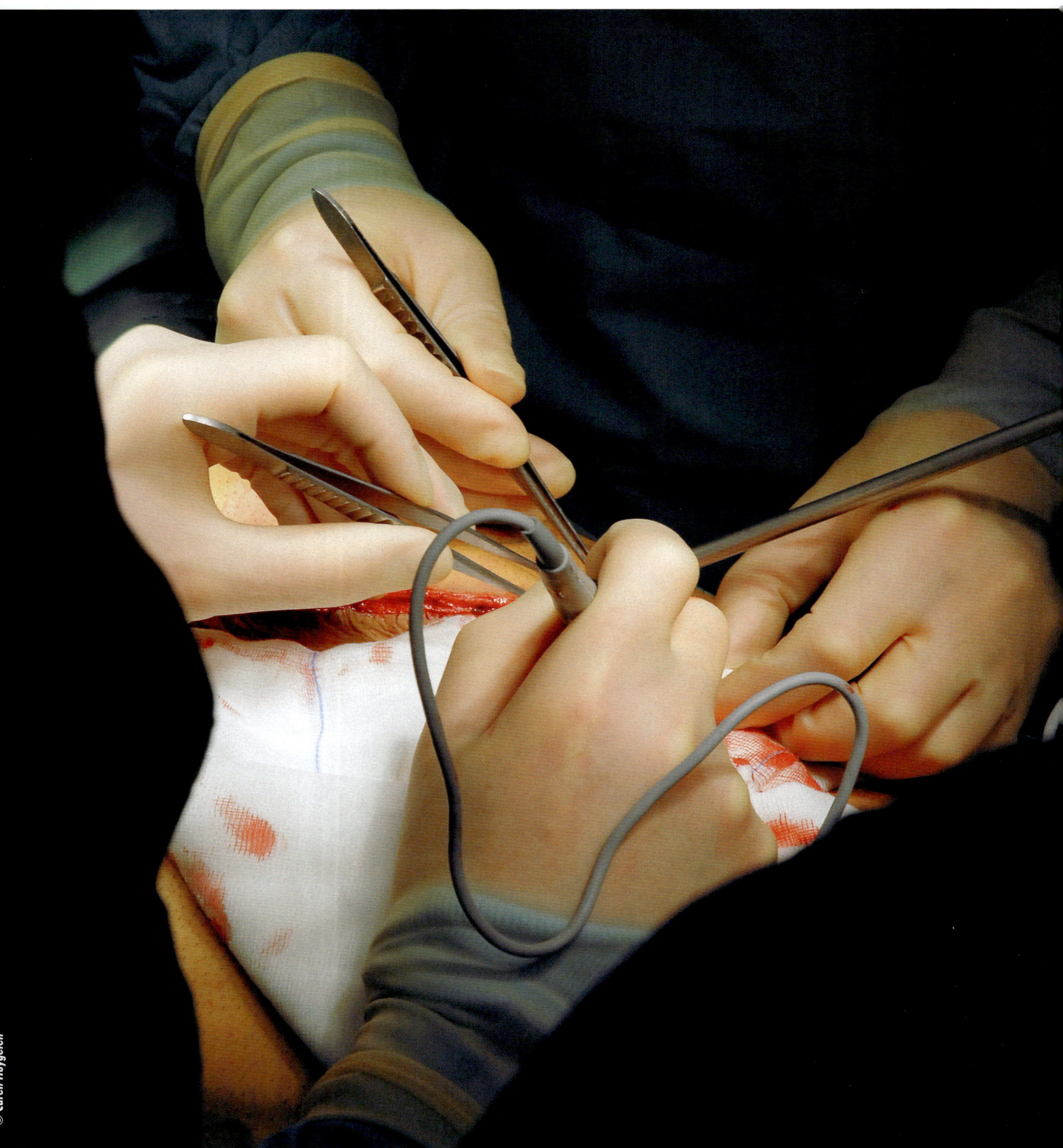

Medical devices: problems and possible solutions

So far, the findings of the report have identified the key medical devices recommended by clinical guidelines for each of the 15 global high-burden diseases and disabilities. In addition, the problems and potential solutions to choosing and using medical devices, and directing medical device innovation, have been highlighted. As explained in the Section 4, medical device activities were categorized in this way (i.e. choosing and using medical devices and medical device innovation) because these categories cover the processes and stages involved in the agenda to improve access to appropriate medical devices, and are directly or indirectly associated with its crucial 4 components—availability, accessibility, appropriateness, and affordability.

5

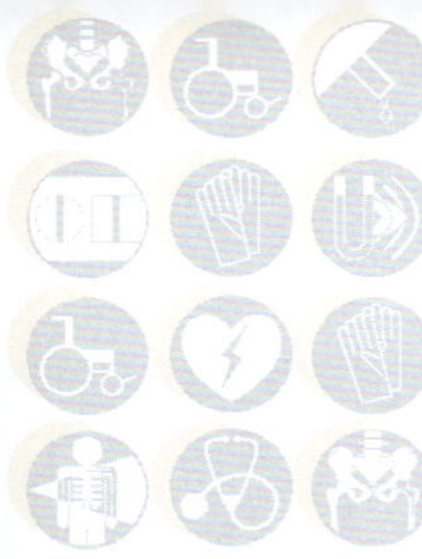

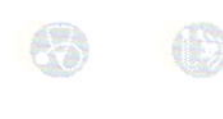

5.1 Choosing medical devices

Choosing a medical device is complex and requires a transparent process based on information, reason, evidence, assessment of public health needs, and a prioritization process. Choosing medical devices without considering the need to improve individual and public health, can lead to inappropriate use or non-use of medical devices and a waste of financial resources. These factors have negative consequences in both industrialized and developing countries. A case in point is the finding that the Netherlands carries out only 17 000 positron emission tomography (PET) scans a year, despite having purchased 24 scanners with an overall capacity to produce nearly three times as many—a possible example of procurement without regard for needs assessment, cost-effectiveness, priorities, and allocation of resources *(117)*.

Diagnostic imaging offers another example of overspending on unneeded devices (and unneeded diagnostic procedures). WHO estimates that high-tech diagnostic imaging is required only in the 20% to 30% of medical cases worldwide in which clinical examination alone is not sufficient to make a correct diagnosis: "Of those cases that require diagnostic imaging, some 80% to 90% of diagnostic problems can generally be solved using basic X-ray and/or ultrasound examinations". Without proper management of demand through needs assessment, adequate procurement and other prerequisites, WHO concludes, "it will be difficult for health-care providers to contain the burgeoning costs *(78)*."

However, with several thousand manufacturers worldwide producing a multitude of medical devices every day, and with distributors and catalogues describing the merits of so many "new and better" devices to potential users, it is understandable that choosing which device to acquire has become a difficult task for ministries of health, regional health authorities and managers of health-care facilities. Lack of professional technical advice from a medical device specialist also contributes to these difficulties. But choosing, and more importantly choosing judiciously, is essential in both high- and low-resource settings.

Assuming that funds to procure medical devices are limited, this report has already shown and discussed the steps required to make rational decisions that are based on public health needs (see Box 3.1 for a stepwise approach to public health needs).

5.1.1 Barriers to choosing medical devices

Major obstacles to rational choosing of a medical device include fascination with technology, aggressive marketing, high costs, and inadequate information about the device. These barriers are discussed in detail below.

Lack of information

The decision to purchase a particular medical device is based on a perceived need that the device will fill. Rational choosing of a medical device will therefore call for information about the need and the extent to which a given device, or category of device, will meet that need.

Lack of adequate information at any step in this sequence or failure to adopt a rational, logical assessment of needs is clearly a barrier to choosing devices likely to achieve a positive health outcome.

A recent report notes that much of the general health-care spending is devoted to activities that do not improve health, and far too little investment is devoted to better understanding the relative advantages among various intervention choices *(118)*. This gap in knowledge about what approaches deliver the best results will only be compounded as the pace of technology development quickens. This publication depicts "a lack of high-quality data" which might have provided evidence for making choices and decisions about devices, particularly devices carrying a significant degree of risk. Patients are asking their doctors for the newest technologies and many physicians do not know where to turn for the latest evidence-based information.

For example, for hospitals deliberating whether to offer cutting-edge technology, such as expensive proton therapy to their patients, there is no evidence available to support improved clinical outcomes over conventional radiation modalities, and no randomized controlled trials making the appropriate comparisons are planned. The problem is compounded by the fact that traditional radiotherapy systems are available at one fifth to one thirtieth of the price of the newer, more expensive systems. Physicians may urge procurement of the high-tech equipment, but they lack the full picture of cost-effectiveness *(28)*.

The lack of objective evaluation and information concerns not only the high-cost, high-tech medical equipment but also the daily supplies and devices that keep a health-care facility running.

However, there are several sources of information that provide that information. Regulatory bodies, such as the FDA in the United States and the Medicines and Healthcare products Regulatory Agency (MHRA) in the United Kingdom, provide information about medical devices but it is generally limited to information needed for market approval, and concerns safety and efficacy of performance during testing rather than effectiveness of a device in actual use. Furthermore, the main function of regulatory authorities is not to seek the comparative data needed for procurement decisions but rather to ensure that a device complies with the statutory requirements for safety, performance, and efficacy.

In addition to national authorities, advisory bodies such as the National Institute for Health and Clinical Excellence (NICE) in the United Kingdom and National Center for Health Technology Excellence (CENETEC) in Mexico also provide evidence on medical devices, with an emphasis on cost-effectiveness.

A second factor limiting the availability of information is that innovative medical devices are usually evaluated for efficacy in relatively small clinical trials—generally too small to identify uncommon complications. While randomized controlled trials are the golden standard for clinical evaluation of pharmaceuticals, use of a placebo or other comparator—a feature of randomized clinical trials for pharmaceuticals—may be impracticable or even unethical in the case of medical devices, particularly implantable devices. One consequence, at least in Europe, according to a recent review of regulatory policies in four large European countries, is that "estimates of the efficacy or even cost-effectiveness of innovative technologies are often still vague" *(119)*.

Another factor hampering availability of information relates to pre-market clinical trials of devices. Normally, to ensure that trial conditions reflect the use of devices by a wide range of users, the clinicians participating in the trials should not be biased by having extensive experience in using the devices and should not be aware of shortcomings in the devices. However, the clinicians participating in a pre-market clinical trial of a device tend to be "well trained in using the device and alert to its possible limitations, and patients are carefully selected for a limited set of medical indications" Once the device is in widespread use by less-skilled or less-trained practitioners and on a broader population of patients, "adverse effects can show up that were not apparent prior to marketing" *(120)*.

Fascination with technology

Fascination with science and technology can blind decision-makers to the need for an objective appraisal based on logic and common sense. Sometimes the mere fact that a particular technology exists appears to be a more important factor in the purchasing decision than its contribution to the care patients receive and their well-being.

In recent years, however, managers of health-care facilities, particularly in high-resource countries, have become reluctant to buy expensive medical equipment. A finding of a recent review by *The Economist* documents this trend: "The proliferation of machinery such as fancy scanners, once applauded, is now criticized as a main cause of runaway health costs. National health systems, private insurers and others who hold the purse strings increasingly demand that innovation be linked to economic value and improved health outcomes" *(25)*.

Deference to personal preference

Over time, health professionals, particularly surgeons, tend to develop preferences for specific brands of devices they use frequently. These preferences can be perfectly legitimate and are often of critical importance to the successful outcome of a clinical procedure. As an industry official notes, the manipulative skill of a clinician with a particular device, such as a surgical instrument or vascular catheter, can influence the outcome of a procedure and that skill can in turn be influenced by the familiar "feel" of a device which the clinician is in the habit of using. Understandably, such "physician-preferred items" have over the years acquired a special status that few hospital managers would challenge. Less legitimate are the special favoured relationships that clinicians may develop with vendors of specific brands of devices—relationships that can run counter to objectivity and concern for health outcomes, ethical codes and professional integrity *(121–124)*.

Preferred items often include expensive devices (implantable pacemakers, cardio-defibrillators, joint implants, coronary stents, and so on) that can account for more than 50% of a hospital's expenditures on medical supplies (which in turn are estimated to account for about 6% of a hospital's total expenditures) *(28, 125, 126)*. In the United States, some health-care facilities are targeting physician's preferences for cost-containment efforts *(28)*. In the end, though, and from the perspective of this report, more important than cost or the manner in which a device is chosen, is the extent to which it will fulfil a fully assessed need for a specific health outcome.

Personal preference can also dictate choices of medical devices in the less developed countries. For example, a student from a resource-limited country, may leave to study medicine in the United States or Europe and during this study period may have learned to work with costly, complex medical devices. On returning to the home country to work in a hospital, the newly graduated physician may wish to offer patients the potential benefits of the complex technology—and of the experience acquired in using it. He or she may then pressure the hospital management to purchase equipment without regard for the need it could fulfil or the overall public health benefit it could bring in its new setting.

Table 5.1 Total health-care expenditure and expenditure on medical technology

Country	Population (1 000)	THE (€ Bn)	THE/GDP	THE per capita (€)	EMT (€ Bn)	EMT per capita (€)	EMT/THE	PMT (€ BN)	Trade balance
Austria	8 233	25,0	9.8%	3.032	1,76	213,77	7.0%	1,79	+
Belgium	10 479	30,5	9.8%	2.911	2,80	267,20	9.2%	1,70	−
Bulgaria	7 699	1,6	6.5%	214	0,13	16,24	7.6%	0,05	−
Cyprus	773	0,8	5.4%	1.027	0,04	52,67	5.1%	0,04	−
Czech Republic	10 221	7,1	7.2%	692	0,54	53,28	7.7%	0,47	−
Denmark	5 416	18,8	8.6%	3.466	1,30	240,03	6.9%	2,20	+
Estonia	1 344	0,6	4.2%	415	0,10	72,36	17.4%	0,06	−
Finland	5 246	11,8	7.1%	2.249	0,53	101,03	4.5%	0,85	+
France	60 873	190,1	10.7%	3.123	10,06	165,26	5.3%	9,44	−
Germany	82 466	238,3	10.4%	2.890	20,20	244,95	8.5%	25,91	+
Greece	11 104	22,9	9.4%	2.061	0,78	70,67	3.4%	0,01	−
Hungary	10 087	6,6	7.4%	653	0,54	53,77	8.2%	0,46	−
Ireland	4 131	12,0	7.5%	2.912	0,41	98,61	3.4%	5,95	+
Italy	58 135	132,4	9.0%	2.278	6,20	106,65	4.7%	2,59	−
Latvia	2 288	0,7	4.4%	306	0,09	37,40	12.2%	0,03	−
Lithuania	3 394	1,2	5.0%	349	0,13	38,24	11.0%	0,09	−
Luxembourg	455	2,5	7.4%	5.386	0,06	128,13	2.4%	0,06	−
Malta	406	0,4	7.9%	984	0,03	66,75	6.8%	0,03	−
Netherlands	16 320	44,4	8.5%	2.721	2,50	153,02	5.6%	3,04	+
Norway	4 661	21,9	8.2%	4.699	1,04	222,63	4.7%	0,80	−
Poland	38 161	15,0	5.6%	394	1,20	31,45	8.0%	0,62	−
Portugal	10 563	15,1	9.8%	1.431	0,72	68,16	4.8%	0,44	−
Romania	21 588	3,8	3.8%	174	0,17	7,91	4.6%	0,03	−
Slovakia	5 387	2,7	6.1%	499	0,24	44,45	8.9%	0,15	−
Slovenia	2 007	2,3	7.6%	1.150	0,21	102,94	9.0%	0,16	−
Spain	43 398	74,4	7.7%	1.714	6,00	138,26	8.1%	3,67	−
Sweden	9 030	25,9	8.4%	2.865	1,38	152,82	5.3%	1,77	+
Switzerland	7 484	34,2	11.0%	4.568	1,68	223,97	4.9%	5,06	+
United Kingom	60 227	147,0	7.7%	2.441	11,75	195,10	8.0%	11,94	+
EUROPE	501 575	1.089,8	8.5%	2.173	72,57	144,69	6.8%	79,43	+
United States	296 410	1511,0	15.3%	5.098	97,96	330,49	6.5%		−

PMT = Production of MT | THE = Total Healthcare Expenditure (total personal expenditure on healthcare + total expenditure on collective services + investment into medical facilities).
EMT = Expenditure on Medical Technology | European averages weighted by population size.
Source: OECD. Eucomed Member Associations. Medistat. and Eucomed Calculations. Reproduced with permission.

The cost of medical devices, known and hidden

Mounting health-care costs, to which the growing number of medical devices are making a significant contribution, are increasingly a cause of concern to a growing number of countries, particularly those with ageing populations—with their increased demand for health care. By the turn of this century, medical devices were accounting for an estimated 5–6% of total health expenditures in Europe, the United States, and Japan. In some European countries (see Table 5.1) the proportion was even higher: 8-9% in Belgium, Germany, and Slovakia and 11–12% in Latvia and Lithuania *(127)*.

Public health authorities have begun questioning whether enough attention is being paid to the cost-effectiveness of the health technologies swelling the market in most industrialized countries *(126)*. Most industrialized countries have cost-containment measures for medicines in place but very few have cost-containment measures for medical devices.

Low-income countries have their particular problems.[1] To take an extreme example, an MRI unit, costing anywhere from US$ 2 million to US$ 8 million *(28, 129)* is likely to be beyond the means of a low-income country. A multi-vault proton therapy system, with a cost of US$ 150 million, would require the entire annual health expenditure of some countries . Even a standard anaesthesia machine costing in the order of US$ 5000 or in vitro diagnostic equipment at more than US$ 250 000 is likely to strain the health system budgets of a low-resource country *(28)*.

Furthermore, the cost of acquiring a medical device, particularly a complex device, is usually only the tip of the financial iceberg. Costs of accessory options, years of warranty, logistics of delivery, installation procedures and recurrent costs for maintenance, spare parts, consumables, reagents for diagnostic kits, and training can amount to more than 80% of the total cost of a device (see Figure 5.1) *(87, 130, 131)*.

---

1   See http://www.who.int/countries/en/, accessed 19 July 2010.

Figure 5.1 The hidden costs of medical devices

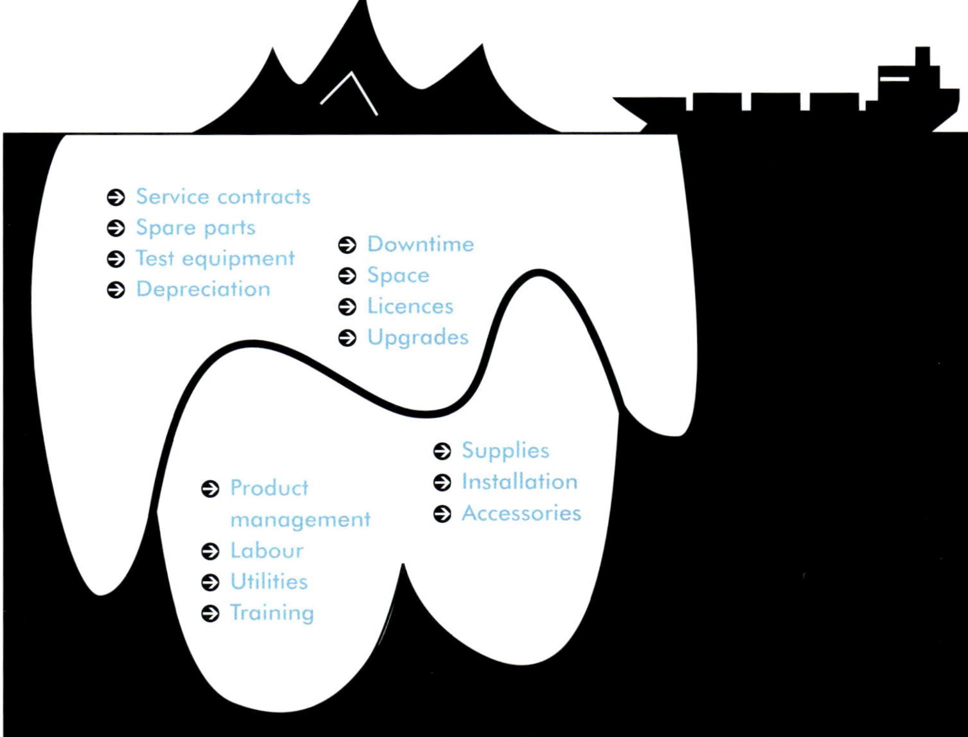

Source: Adapted from Cheng *(41).*

To some extent, the difficulty for countries may be compounded by their cost management systems. The health budgets of almost all developing countries have a line item for medicines but very few have them for medical devices, which often remain an unplanned, unbudgeted expenditure.

On a broader scale, inconsistency of pricing can complicate the procurement process. A study in Benin, for example, compared the prices paid by the Ministry of Health with those paid by private health-care facilities for 10 selected devices marketed by 10 device companies: the results showed that between 1998 and 2008 the Ministry had been paying between two and six times more for these devices than the private health-care facilities *(132)*. Generally speaking, international bidding can keep prices down, as can procurement from official company distributors rather than from distributors, who can be part of a long chain of middlemen, each taking a share of the profit.

Lack of a single nomenclature

There are three key areas where a lack of standardization negatively affects the rational choice of medical device procurement—regulation, standards, and nomenclature. Harmonization towards regulation and standards are briefly mentioned in Chapter 5.1.2. However, as something so basic poses such problems for appropriately choosing medical devices, lack of a single nomenclature is discussed in detail here.

The *PMD* project used the GHTF definition of medical devices for the purposes of this report. However there are a number of different nomenclatures currently being used throughout world, such as the *Global Medical Device Nomenclature (GMDN)*, [2] the *Universal Medical Device Nomenclature System (UMDNS)*,[3] the *Standard ISO 9999* (a classification system for assistive products that are used by people with disabilities)[4] and the *Harmonized System of the World Customs Organization*.[5]

In addition, other nomenclatures have been forged by individual countries (Japan, Mexico, Norway, the Russian Federation, and many others) or by national or international organizations (e.g. Médecins Sans Frontières, UNICEF), essentially for their own specific purposes.

Since each nomenclature identifies a given medical device by a different name or code, the current patchwork of multiple nomenclatures defeats the primary purpose of a nomenclature, at least on a global level, namely to provide a universally accepted means of identifying every medical device on the market according to its intended use. A universal nomenclature system could improve several areas related to medical devices, as described below.

As there are several nomenclatures currently in use around the world, a procurement manager, health official, national regulatory authority, hospital inventory manager, marketing manager, or product vendor is likely to find it difficult to exchange information about a medical device—including reports of adverse events associated with its use—with any person in any country not using the same nomenclature system. Even within a single country, a single coding or nomenclature system can be a valuable asset, but which is not overseen by any regulatory agencies. In the United States, for example, the FDA is considering whether a unique device identification system is warranted given its potential "to help reduce medical errors, facilitate recalls, identify incompatibility with devices or potential allergic reactions, improve inventory control, improve reimbursement, and reduce product counterfeiting" *(89)*.

Clearly, the lack of a single, globally accepted international nomenclature is an important barrier to choosing a medical device.

Marketing practices

Collusion and corruption

One barrier to making rational choices about medical devices is collusion between physicians and vendors of medical devices. The existing evidence suggests that the practice is widespread in both industrialized and developing countries *(123, 124, 133)*. A code of conduct for both the medical device industry and health authorities is necessary.

---

2   http://www.gmdnagency.org, accessed 13 July 2010.
3   https://www.ecri.org/Products/Pages/UMDNS.aspx, accessed 13 July 2010.
4   http://www.iso.org/iso/iso_catalogue/catalogue_tc/catalogue_detail.htm?csnumber=38894, accessed 13 July 2010.
5   http://www.wcoomd.org/home_hsoverviewboxes.htm, accessed 13 July 2010.

Several manufacturers and industry umbrella organizations, however, do have ethical codes governing the relationship between a manufacturer and health-care providers. Many also have watchdog bodies (including non-industry representatives) that monitor manufacturers' compliance with the codes.

Transparency International, a global civil society organization set up to combat corruption, ranks procurement of drugs and medical equipment fourth on a list of seven processes that carry a high risk of corruption. Experts interviewed by this organization alleged that health ministry officials and hospital administrators "inflate the cost of medical equipment in collusion with private suppliers and share the non-reported difference, which can be as much as five times the true cost" *(122)*. Large public health-care programmes in the United States lose 5–10% of their budget through this form of overpayment *(122)*.

Failings of post-market surveillance systems

For a hospital or clinic in the process of deciding what device to buy, one important factor is to know how safe and effective a given device is in actual use. Post-market surveillance is a way to follow-up on the safety and effectiveness of a device.

Manufacturers are required to undertake post-market surveillance for all medical devices they have placed on the market. Regulatory authorities require the manufacturers to report to them unexpected problems of safety or usage detected by the surveillance system. However, there are several shortcomings of post-market surveillance systems and adverse event reporting for medical devices.

One is the fact that adverse event reporting relies on a passive process, namely, receiving reports of adverse events as they occur and are reported. This procedure is notoriously unreliable and leaves a large proportion of adverse events underreported. In the United States, the FDA has a mandatory adverse event reporting system for medical device users, but in fact receives far more reports from manufacturers than users. A similar surveillance system is run by the MHRA in the United Kingdom. In practice, few users of medical devices report incidents to regulators or manufacturers (a study commissioned by the United States Congress in the 1980s found that less than

1% of adverse events linked to the use of medical devices were reported to the FDA by hospitals *(120)*.

Another weakness of post-market surveillance is that it generally does not provide data on the number of devices at risk for a given adverse event: it is thus impossible to calculate the incidence rate of such events and to balance the known benefits of a device with its safety profile. Manufacturers' monitoring systems are closely, but not exclusively, based on incidence rates derived from estimates of numbers of devices remaining in service. But in practice these systems suffer from a degree of imprecision because of differences in the average service life of a device. A failing of both adverse event reporting and post-market surveillance reporting systems is that there is no reliable system in place for rigorous follow-up and public reporting of adverse events associated with the use of medical devices (e.g. high risk implanted devices like implantable pacemakers). The current system depends on isolated registries, frequently supported by industry or professional associations, and on voluntary reporting by vigilant, experienced individual clinicians.

In 2006, the GHTF initiated the National Competent Authority Report (NCAR) programme to standardize and facilitate adverse event reporting by manufacturers to competent authorities.

Counterfeiting

Counterfeiting of medical products can also defeat the purpose of rationally choosing these products. There is evidence that the practice is growing. In 2007, 1500 counterfeiting incidents—mainly medicines—were detected worldwide, roughly 20% more than in the previous year and ten times as many as in 2000, according to a WHO report submitted to the Sixty-first World Health Assembly in 2008 *(134)*. Counterfeit medical products, including medical devices and medicines, have been detected in most of WHO's 193 Member States, the report notes. They include medical devices, such as contact lenses, condoms, surgical mesh and self-monitoring blood glucose test strips *(134)*.

Deficiencies of clinical guidelines

Clinical guidelines, specific care pathways, and clinical protocols are currently available to identify the medical devices on the basis of clinical need, evidence, and best practices. Clinical guidelines have been defined by WHO as "systematically developed evidence-based statements which assist providers, recipients and other stakeholders to make informed decisions about appropriate health interventions" *(135)*. Over the past decade, the quest for evidence-based information has expanded in most areas of health care and with it, the production of clinical guidelines *(136)*. Health insurance companies, international and national health organizations, professional associations and many others, are contributing to the large number of clinical guidelines. The proliferation of clinical guidelines also reflects an increasing effort by health authorities to limit health-care costs and to put pressure on clinicians to abide by the most cost-effective, best practices.

Yet, for many health-care providers, guidelines have not become essential reading *(135)*. A study exploring the barriers to guideline adherence identified six common factors related to physicians' knowledge, attitudes and behaviour: lack of awareness by physicians of the existence of specific guidelines, disagreement with guideline recommendations, scepticism over the feasibility of applying guidelines successfully, lack of familiarity with the content of guidelines, failure to consider health outcomes that could result from applying guidelines, and resistance to changing personal practice *(137)*.

However, part of the problem is also the clinical guidelines themselves. Some of these guidelines, care pathways or protocols do not specify which medical devices should be used in performing a clinical procedure. In addition, assistive devices are not mentioned in clinical guidelines. These devices make up a large and extremely varied category of devices, used to assist people with functional disability *(32)*.

With so many national and international associations and organizations issuing guidelines, there are inevitably multiple recommendations on the same topic, each based on different premises and different types of evidence *(137)*. Several guidelines make recommendations that are not conclusive or do not indicate the source of the evidence on which they are based *(135)*. And those that do indicate sources often include recommendations—about half in one

review study—that are not based on high-quality evidence *(136)*.

Attempts have been made to improve clinical guidelines. For example, the AGREE (Appraisal of Guidelines Research & Evaluation) Collaboration, formed in 1998 and funded by the European Union, established a quality assessment instrument to help improve the quality and effectiveness of clinical practice guidelines.

Another problem with clinical guidelines is the difficulty of keeping them up to date. Medical devices tend to change rapidly with the growing pace of technological innovation, as do other elements of a clinical procedure with advances in clinical state-of-the-art practice. Finally, guidelines may be affected by bias because of specific interest of developers *(138)*.

5.1.2 Possible solutions to overcoming these barriers

Given the wide range of key obstacles to the rational choice of medical devices, there is an equally long list of possible solutions to overcome each barrier. However, in the interests of pragmatism, the discussion below focuses on the main areas involved in any possible solution—rational decision-making (including more useful clinical guidelines and development of a single nomenclature for medical devices), public health need, cost containment, and improvement of marketing practices.

However, before moving on to these solutions, it is important to mention how "harmonization" of some of the factors involved in choosing medical devices is helping the current situation—regulation and standards.

The diversity of regulatory practices from one country to another largely stems from historical and cultural differences. Fostering convergence of regulatory practices is the main objective of the GHTF, whose five study groups of experts have produced guidelines and recommendations on many aspects of medical device regulation *(139–143)*. Together, these guidelines constitute a framework that any country can use to align its regulatory system with those of other countries.

WHO defines standards as "documented agreements containing technical specifications or other precise criteria to be used consistently as rules, guidelines or definitions of characteristics, to ensure that materials, products, processes and services are fit for their purpose" *(3)*. However, there are few standards against which compliance with reliability, safety, efficacy and quality of medical devices can be measured. Several international organizations—such as the International Organization for Standardization (ISO),[6] The International Electrotechnical Commission (IEC), and the International Telecommunication Union (ITU)—have developed international standards that are widely used in the medical device community. The GHTF urges national regulatory authorities to recognize and apply these standards.

Rational decision-making

Decisions about which medical devices to procure should result from a rational process that takes into account the key factors on which choices must be based—public health need, cost, cost-effectiveness, and likely health outcome. This report has suggested a stepwise approach to choosing medical devices (see Box 3.1), which could be used as a practical tool for selecting the priority medical devices best suited to the management of priority health problems.

When choosing a medical device, a health-care facility or public health authority in any setting should make their decision based on answers to such questions as: What clinical need will the device fulfil? Does the need correspond to accepted health-care practice? Will the device improve public health? Is the cost of the device justified by the need? Will paying that cost divert funds needed for other, higher-priority acquisitions? Is it a priority in this particular setting? Has evidence of adequate safety and effectiveness been obtained? Is the device appropriate to the level of health care (primary, secondary, tertiary) at which it will be used and to the likely availability of resources for upkeep, maintenance, repair, and other ancillary requirements? Is training being provided? Is the physical infrastructure adequate?

Such questions, most experts believe, are best answered by a team consisting of several specialists— biomedical engineers, medical staff, nursing staff and financial staff mandated to make choices on the strength of a rational process that gives priority to health needs of the target population. Where possible, the procurement process should be managed by a team representing the different functions carried out within the health-care facility, which is aware of the budgetary limitations constraining their choices. The size and composition of the team will depend on the size and nature of the health-care facility. However, ideally, a biomedical engineer should be part of the team to ensure the precise identification of devices meeting specifications of medical device design, structure, and performance.

Making clinical guidelines more useful

Several improvements could make clinical guidelines more useful for rationally choosing medical devices. A guideline could, for example, take the form of a flowchart or decisional algorithm—a care pathway— which takes the user through a series of steps, or choices, leading to a list identifying precisely the devices (or medicines or other resources) needed for the management of a given disease or disability. And in recommending devices, or combinations of devices for a given procedure, the protocols ideally urge readers to consider whether the required technical skills and supportive infrastructure are available for safe, effective use of the recommended devices.

The care pathway could recommend medical devices ranked by the proportion of cases in which it might be used by a given health-care facility or setting, thereby allowing procurement decisions to give priority to those devices likely to be used most often. Such guidelines, care pathways and protocols could be used in every country by health-care facilities at any level of the health system—primary (district hospital), secondary (provincial hospital), or tertiary (central or regional hospital)—and for any clinical condition, however mild or severe.

Developing a single nomenclature

A universally accepted and adopted nomenclature system would greatly enhance rational decision-making for choosing medical devices. WHO could facilitate the development of such a system.

---

6   International Organization for Standardization (ISO) (http://www.iso.org, accessed 17 July 2010).

Public health need

Almost all relatively complex medical devices on the market today have been made, and designed for use, in high-resource countries. Their usability in low-resource settings is limited. For health-care providers in both industrialized and developing countries, the choice of medical devices must take into account the potential health impact of a device as shown in the stepwise approach discussed in Section 3.

Health technology assessment (HTA) is an approach which evaluates clinical effectiveness, cost, and outcome. Broadly speaking, an HTA of a medical device would cover its technical properties, safety, efficacy (in controlled conditions), effectiveness in actual use (preferably in patient outcomes), functionality, economic impact, and social, legal, ethical, or political impact. HTA is currently used by ministers of health, health-care payers and providers, professional health associations, hospitals and other health-care facilities, health maintenance organizations, health insurance companies, government officials, and law-makers.

Factors that HTA should take into account in assessing the cost-effectiveness of a technology are listed in a so-called "PICO" framework: the characteristics of the *Population* in which the technology will be used, the *Intervention* used, its *Comparator*, and its expected *Outcome*. However, different countries and users tend to develop their own specific modalities for carrying out the assessments. The United Kingdom's National Health Service R&D Health Technology Assessment Programme defines HTA as a means of answering four questions: Does the technology work? Who needs it? What does it cost? How does it compare with alternative technologies *(144)*?

HTA has its supporters and opponents. Some see the growing complexity and capabilities of medical devices as strengthening the need for HTA. Others express resistance to the practice for reasons that include its cost in time, effort, and money. Some observers believe that the HTA process should itself be the subject of an assessment. Is there evidence, they ask, that HTA is itself cost-effective? Does it, in fact, benefit health-care systems to the extent claimed by its proponents? Yet others point out that health technology assessment is an evolving and imperfect science, that many of its methods are still controversial and that often its results will differ depending on the models, cost assumptions, and other variables that are used for the assessment.

There are also those who are unwilling to make the changes in their clinical practice that HTA might call for. And, of course, among those infatuated with technology, many expect that "new is better" and see no reason for systematic assessment of a technology that has a potential for some benefit, however marginal or poorly substantiated *(145)*.

Health technology assessments reports are used in governments for decision-making such as the Canadian Agency for Drugs and Technologies in Health (CADTH), and Danish Centre for Health Technology Assessment (DACEHTA), Swedish Council on health technology Assessment in Health Care (SBU), NICE in the United Kingdom, and CENETEC in Mexico.

Another approach to making information available about the potential value of a device would be to create an international repository or clearing house where all the evidence concerning a medical device could be gathered by a body such as WHO and made available on a dedicated web site for consultation by all interested parties, including procurement managers *(10)*.

Containing costs

In assessing prices of medical devices, a health-care facility's procurement team might use consumer reports, suppliers' catalogues, and other sources of information. To limit costs and leverage competitive pricing, the team could benchmark device prices or develop a "formulary" of preferred suppliers to limit marketing pressure from an unlimited number of suppliers.

Pooled or bulk procurement arrangements can also limit costs and are used by international agencies such as UNICEF and WHO for procurement of devices on behalf of a number of Member States. In some regions, countries have formed groupings for pooled purchasing: an example is the Gulf Cooperation Council that brings together the six Arab states of the Persian Gulf *(146)*. In some countries, several hospitals or clinics have started using bulk purchasing mechanisms, such as "integrated delivery networks", where a single team manages procurement for several health-care providers in a given locality *(147)*.

In addition, reference price lists of medical devices used in a selected number of countries could be made available publicly in order to facilitate price benchmarking. Key medical devices required for the management of a selected number of high-burden diseases could serve as reference products for price benchmarking. Benchmarking includes setting purchasing prices, operational and maintenance indicators, as well as other costs required for acquisition and for the technical life-cycle of the medical devices.

Improving marketing practices

There are many possible solutions that could be suggested for improving marketing practices but for the purposes of this report, only a few are selected.

Improved regulation

Even within the approximately one third of WHO member states that have some regulatory framework, implementation of regulatory oversight is highly variable in efficacy and comprehensiveness. Ideally, in the future, no medical device could be used anywhere without having acquired market approval from a fully operational regulatory system. For this to happen, every country without a regulatory system could begin to put in place such a system at a rate and to an extent compatible with its resources and public health priorities. In addition, a mechanism could be devised whereby devices accorded market approval by a country with an established regulatory system are deemed to fulfil regulatory requirements in countries not yet possessing a fully operational regulatory system.

Tackling corruption

Efforts at combating corruption have also produced innovative tactics. Making information available, for example, has been shown to reduce losses due to corruption. A Transparency International report showed that the variation across hospitals in prices paid for medical supplies dropped by 50% in Argentina after the Ministry began to disseminate information about how much hospitals were paying for their supplies. Purchase prices for the monitored items immediately fell by an average of 12% *(122)*.

Other measures to combat corruption include procurement guidelines, codes of conduct for operators in the health sector, and transparency and monitoring procedures.

Tackling counterfeiting

Eucomed, an umbrella organization for European medical device manufacturers, has called on its members "to incorporate features in products and packaging to distinguish genuine from counterfeit products" *(148)*. It also calls, among other things, for a "zero-tolerance public policy" including calling for laws which would make it easier to prosecute counterfeiters and carry heavier penalties for offenders. For its part, the European Commission is considering adding traceability requirements to its list of essential requirements for medical devices *(149)*. In November 2008, IMPACT,[7] an anti-counterfeit coalition, extended its mandate, previously focused on medicines, to include medical devices.

5.2 Using medical devices

For the sake of clarity, the following discussion on the barriers to using medical devices assumes that a proper choice of a medical device has been made and that the problem now is whether or not it will be properly used, and if not, why not.

Logically, for a device to be used, it must be usable. As expert research and reflection over the past two decades have made clear, the main barrier to usability of a medical device is the inappropriateness of its design in relation to the context of its intended use *(150)*. And from a usability or context-dependent perspective, the onus is to a certain extent on the choosers to select a device likely to fit the context in which it will be used. But the onus is also—and perhaps especially—on manufacturers to design their devices to be contextually appropriate.

5.2.1 Barriers to using medical devices

Although discussed under different headings below, barriers to using medical devices are largely interrelated and stem from a mix of factors. The relative importance of each factor will vary with the context—geographical, social, cultural, economic,

---

7   http://www.who.int/impact/en/ (accessed 13 July 2010).

demographic, medical, reimbursement—in which a medical device will be used.

Donations

Donations of medical devices, particularly complex equipment, often do not match the recipient's needs. Seldom does the recipient of a donated medical device participate in the selection of the device. In this sense, donations constitute an insidious barrier to choosing appropriate medical devices.

Many low-resource countries rely heavily on donations of medical devices to equip what health-care facilities they have. In fact, some acquire nearly 80% of their health-care equipment in the form of donations from international bodies or foreign governments. Only 10–30% of donated equipment, however, actually becomes operational, according to one estimate *(151)*. A donor may not think of the infrastructure needed to operate medical equipment, or forget or neglect to ship an essential cable or accessory; the equipment may break in shipping, or the staff of the recipient hospital may be unable to install or use the equipment *(131)*.

Donors have drawn criticism for failing to ensure that donated equipment is functional, meets standards of safety and performance, comes with an adequate supply of spare parts and consumables, and is the type of technology that the recipient wants, needs, and is able to use and keep using *(151)*. Donors may supply devices free of charge but leave the recipient to bear the running costs: in countries too poor to bear these costs, the equipment ends up unused. Likewise, some medical device manufacturers have been known to offer expensive devices free of charge to hospitals in high- and low-resource countries, and then recoup the costs from the consumable supplies needed to keep the devices functioning.

The motivation of donors has also been questioned. Keeping their own hospital corridors clear of obsolete equipment and making room for new technologies, while acquiring a good conscience (and perhaps a

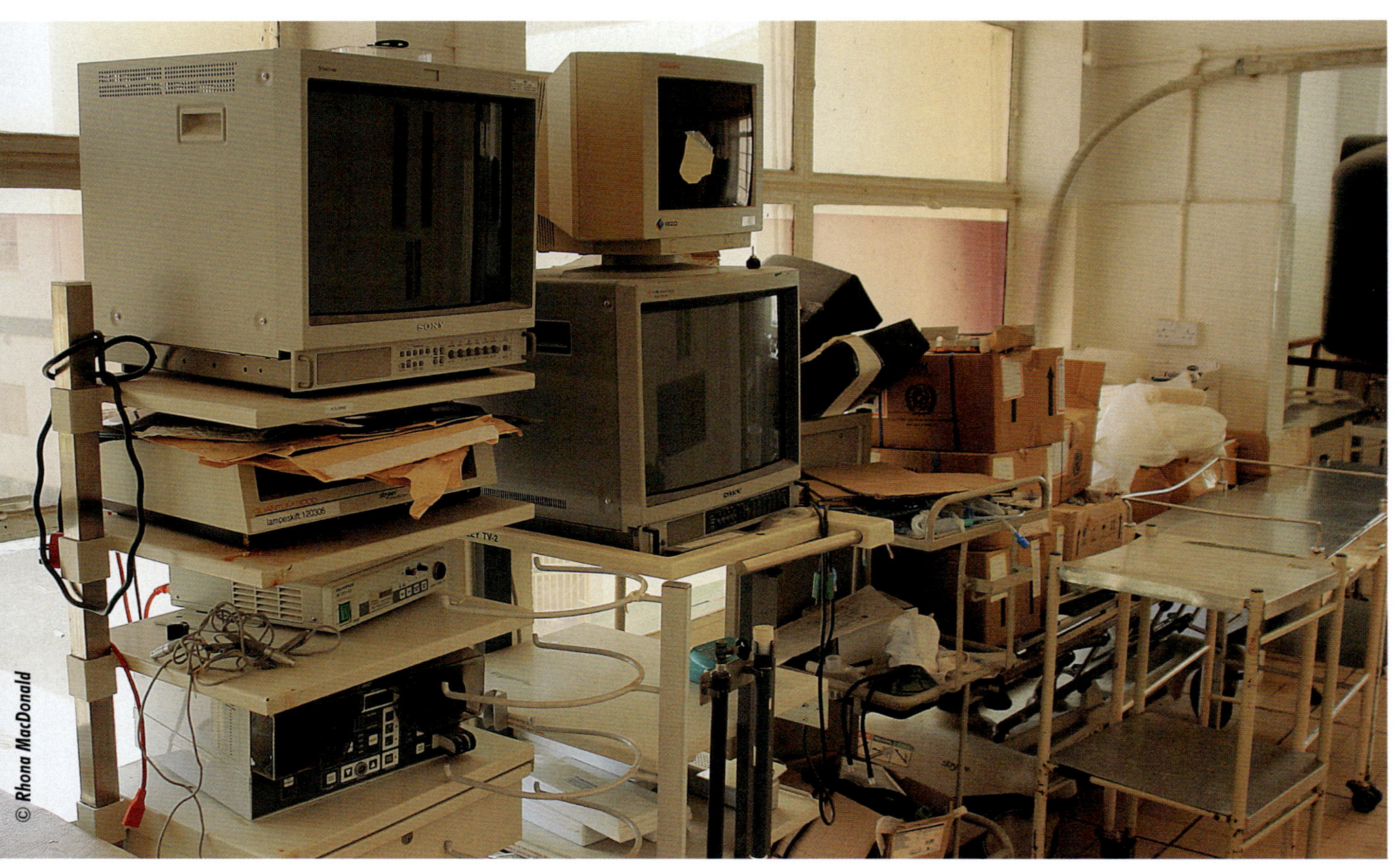

tax reduction), are often-quoted motivations. Some donors elude their responsibility in the belief that for low-resource countries "anything is better than nothing." *(152)*

Recipient countries may contribute to the problem. Recipients do not always assess their needs nor do they invest in the time or resources needed to plan for the functioning of the equipment. Nor do they always take the time and effort to inform prospective donors of their needs. And when they do, they do not always indicate whether they have the resources, human and financial, to install, operate, and maintain the requested equipment.

Used or refurbished equipment is often donated and can also prove problematic. In many cases, such equipment does not work for any significant length of time or when it does, local arrangements for training and accessories are needed to keep it working *(152)*. Since the 1980s, responding to the risks and drawbacks of medical device donations, intergovernmental and nongovernmental organizations, professional medical associations, ministries of health, biomedical engineering associations, and charitable organizations have developed guidelines for donors and recipients of medical devices. A WHO guideline, published in 2000, spells out four core principles of medical device donation *(152)*:

- The donation should benefit the recipient to the maximum extent possible;
- The donation should respect the wishes and authority of the recipient and conform to existing government policies and administrative arrangements;
- If the quality of an item is unacceptable in the donor country, it is also unacceptable as a donation;
- All donations should result from a need expressed by the recipient.

These guidelines are due to be updated soon.

Inappropriate design

Context

Manufacturers are being increasingly called upon to consider contextual factors in designing their medical devices. The context of use is defined as "a

Figure 5.2 A context pyramid

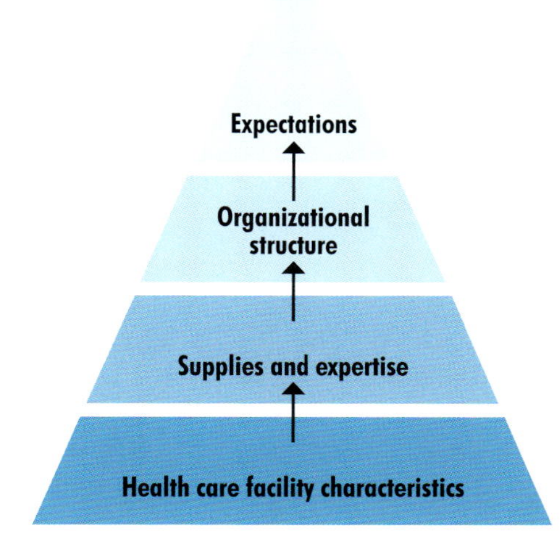

Source: *(150)*.

complex of factors that influence the use of a medical device in a day-to-day working environment" *(150)*. Four layers of contextual factors are distinguished (Figure 5.2). Each of the top three layers is dependent on the layer or layers below it. For example, it is of minimal value to focus on patients' expectations without addressing the adequate training of the health-care personnel operating the device *(150)*.

Contextual factors can be viewed from a variety of perspectives. The user's perspective is important for the design of the medical device *(150)*. Context will also include the type of health-care facility in which the user will use a device. Devices to be used in a health-care facility, for example, are likely to differ in design from those intended for home use. Those devices to be used in a primary health-care centre are likely to differ in design from those to be used in a hospital and so on. If used at home or by people with functioning problems, the design should differ in important respects from the same type of device to be used by trained health-care workers. Table 5.2 shows a variety of devices used in the home and hospital.

Home use

Home use of complex medical devices is increasing. As a result, there are calls for manufacturers to develop their risk assessment with the users in mind.

Table 5.2 Medical devices by purpose, place of use and user

	Medical devices			
Context of use	**Preventive**	**Diagnostic**	**Therapeutic**	**Assistive**
Main users	Health-care professionals or healthy individuals	Health-care professionals or patients	Health-care professionals or patients	Individuals or health-care professionals
Examples of medical devices used in health-care facilities	Surgical gloves, sterilization equipment, disinfectants	Laboratory diagnostic tests, X-ray equipment, MRI, electrocardiogram, stethoscopes, blood gas analysers, endoscopes, tongue depressors, reflex hammers	Orthopaedic implants, surgical equipment, pacemakers, stents, infusion pumps, ventilators, sterile dressings, laparoscopes	Traction devices, patient hoists, hospital beds, operating tables, prostheses, ortheses
Examples of medical devices used in homes	Condoms, gloves, pessary	Pregnancy tests, blood glucose tests, blood pressure meters, telemedicine, cardiac monitoring	Infusion pumps, dialysis equipment, oxygen supply systems, syringes	Crutches, wheelchairs, spectacles, eye lenses, hoists

Patients are "much less able [than professionals] to overcome device limitations [and] there is greater pressure on the designer of a home-health care device to reduce those limitations". The designer "must assume that the user may have physical, perceptual, or cognitive disabilities" *(36)*.

Tailoring medical device design to specific contexts does not necessarily require major changes in design. For example, a kidney dialysis machine intended for home use could be made more user-friendly by incorporating a few elements into its design—a larger, brighter screen, more easily identifiable controls, and perhaps more electronic circuitry to monitor, advise, and protect the user *(16)*.

Low-resource settings

Low-resource settings present a design challenge not only for device manufacturers but also for governments responsible for setting and applying health technology policies aimed at improving or maintaining the health of their populations.

Currently, most medical equipment used in low-resource settings is imported from industrialized countries. About 70% of the more complex devices do not function when they reach their destination in developing countries *(130)*. The main reason is the disparity between the context in which the devices are expected to function, and the context in which they do.

In industrialized countries, for example, there are stable sources of electricity and clean water required by devices to operate correctly. Manufacturers have had little reason to design and produce devices that will function in parts of the world where sources of power are unreliable or non-existent. Inadequate power supply was the single most common cause of medical device failure found by a university training programme that collected data from 33 hospitals in 10 developing countries: nearly a third of equipment failures were due to power problems *(130)*.

In addition, in low-resource settings, medical equipment is likely to face conditions for which it may not have been designed, such as temperature extremes and dusty environments.

High-resource settings

In high-resource settings, the design of medical devices can also be problematic, as the following list of selected examples illustrates.

Faulty operator–interface design of computerized systems for monitoring the life signs of critical-care patients can allow medical staff to miss crucial alarm settings, leading to the death of the patient *(153)*.

Blades used for tracheal intubation are packaged in a way that prevents their rapid removal. Yet the device is frequently used in emergencies that call for urgent action *(154)*.

Many infusion pumps are too complex to ensure correct programming by health practitioners, according to a 2004 study *(155)*. Poor display design can have fatal consequences *(156)*. Small changes in the delivery rate of the pump can be caused by a mobile phone placed on an inadequately protected pump stand *(157)*. Moreover, the multiplicity of different types of infusion pumps can also complicate the task of choosing the right pump for the right indication *(158)*.

A Luer Taper connection is a universal method of joining needles and syringes to small-bore medical tubing. However, the uniformity of Luer Taper connections allows busy health-care personnel to sometimes mistakenly connect a wide range of devices with completely different functions. For example, when the tube from a portable blood-pressure monitoring device is mistakenly connected to a patient's intravenous line, it can cause an air embolism and subsequent death.

On receiving reports of wheelchairs spontaneously driving off curbs and piers whenever a police or fire vehicle or harbour patrol boat operates in the vicinity, an FDA investigation found that the motor controllers of the wheelchairs were sensitive to electromagnetic interference, which released the wheelchair brakes and sent the wheelchairs in random directions *(157)*.

Limited management

Many devices have been procured without a clear medical device management plan of how to maintain them to ensure functionality, safety, accuracy and durability. For example, a recent study conducted in an eastern Mediterranean country showed that from 1996 to 2004 the amount the government spent on repairs of medical devices was more than 2.5 times the amount it would have needed to maintain the equipment by adopting standard annual inspections and management of maintenance contracts *(78)*.

Management of medical devices in high-resource settings is not a simple task either. A single hospital can have thousands of medical devices, with various models of the same type *(16)*. Hence the need for greater standardization, which would not only simplify the use, repair, and servicing of multiple devices but also the integration of several devices used in a single system or network. Lack of standardization is clearly a barrier to using medical devices.

The World Bank estimated that over 50% of medical equipment in developing countries is not maintained and is out of order: "Developing countries could obtain greater returns on their investments in medical devices if they would pay greater attention to ensuring adequate recurrent budget, training of operators and staff and the introduction of good management practices" *(41)*. However, poor use of medical devices in low-resource settings is sometimes a consequence of the lack infrastructure—roads, electrical power, landline and mobile telephones, Internet connectivity—essential for medical devices to be used to their full potential.

In addition, low-income countries often lack not only the funds, but also the experience required to create and run an efficient medical device management system. Efficient procurement, utilization, inventory management, repair and maintenance, and other requisites for proper utilization of medical devices, is difficult without a qualified person to manage a medical device management system. Until such systems are in place, the major barriers to using medical devices will persist. A combination of inadequate planning and inadequate financial resources could explain why one study found that 75% of district hospitals in developing countries had no access to the oxygen needed to operate life-saving ventilators and of those that did, most had only enough for about three months *(159)*.

In addition to the policy choices at health ministry level, appropriate management of medical devices is also the responsibility of the managers of individual health-care facilities, heads of department, biomedical engineers, physicians, and nursing staff. To implant an artificial knee, for example, requires an appropriate aseptic operative setting, with the right surgical instruments, sterile solutions, and standby blood for emergencies, as well as well-trained, qualified staff. Without a management system, such a coordinated deployment of human and material resources would be impossible.

Using even the most basic, commonplace medical devices requires management. For example, inexpensive, disposable plastic syringes—the devices of choice for injections—cannot be safely reused as there is no reliable way of cleaning them. But in some settings, despite their low cost, these disposable devices will be reused, putting patients at risk of infection. Correct waste management procedures are urgently required to lower such risks.

Lack of training

Operating a medical device, even a relatively simple one such as patient hoists *(160)*, requires knowledge and skills. Both are acquired through education, training, and experience. Devices, such as active implantable devices, often call for well-coordinated, well-trained teams of specialists, supporting professionals and laboratory backup staff (for electrophysiology and catheterization, for example). Lack of appropriate health staff training in the use of medical devices may constitute a considerable barrier to using medical devices safely *(155)*.

The relatively high frequency of reported errors in the use of medical devices in industrialized countries points to shortcomings in the training of users. In 2000, for example, the FDA received over 90 000 reports on device-related errors, of which a third involved use-related errors. Use errors in anaesthesiology account for as much as 90% of the deaths and injuries to patients, according to one estimate *(155)*.

Lack of training is not the only cause of use errors. Mistakes often result from a combination of factors such as poor equipment design, poorly written labels and failure to read equipment manuals. A study in 2007 found inadequate training to be the third most common cause of an adverse event linked to a medical device, after use error and inappropriate medical device design *(155)*.

Training in the use of medical devices faces several constraints. One is that acquiring the skills needed to use complex medical devices involves a particularly long learning curve *(155)*. Another is that, unlike many other areas of health care, medical devices tend to have a relatively short commercial life-cycle, on average about 18 months *(39)*, during which new, more technologically advanced models are continually replacing earlier models. A limited number of countries have academic institutions that provide a training curriculum for biomedical engineering. And where practical training is provided, it is usually confined to a very small number of the numerous devices on the market.

Certain working conditions in hospitals or clinics can also hamper proper training. Organizing training sessions for part-time employees (who may, for example, work for only two days a week or only on night shifts) can be problematic. Shift work generally can make training impossible or difficult, with shift handover periods disrupting continuity of training. Lack of standardization, with different models or brands of the same device requiring different operating procedures, can also frustrate attempts at training.

Although medical device manufacturers or distributors may have provided training in the use of their products as part of the procurement contract, a one-time training session is often insufficient to meet the level of competency needed to operate the increasingly complex devices that hospitals are acquiring *(41)*. Technical information, in the form of instruction manuals or direct communication from distributors, could to some extent compensate for failings in user training. But most manuals for imported devices, including those donated by industrialized countries, are not in the language of the receiving country—making them incomprehensible to many health workers. Even the few manuals that are translated into a local language might contain unreliable information due to inaccuracies of translation.

Furthermore, a training curriculum in the use of a device can very rapidly become out-of-date, particularly those targeted at surgeons, device operators, and nurses. *(155)* Hospital administrators may be willing to hire staff and pay for training if potential trainees were available *(130)*. However, in poorer countries, suitable candidates tend to join the "brain drain" exodus towards industrialized countries, which offer more favourable career prospects and more opportunities to acquire skills in using high-tech devices than their home countries. Therefore availability of medical devices, training in their use, and improved work opportunities are important factors for retaining human resources.

The high turnover of medical professionals in developing countries and a constant need for trained staff to replace those who leave for more attractive positions elsewhere pose massive problems to health-care delivery *(41)*. A recent WHO report points out that sub-Saharan Africa is the region most severely affected by shortage of trained staff to operate medical devices: with 11% of the world's population and 24% of the world's disease burden, it has only 3% of the world's health workers *(109)*.

Maintenance problems

Inadequate maintenance is the main reason why so much medical equipment is lying idle in developing countries. Proper maintenance requires a budget, industry technicians for specific maintenance, and ready access to spare parts. But most of all, adequate maintenance requires properly trained staff to order the correct spare parts, install them properly and, generally, to perform the regular tasks required to keep a medical device in working condition.

Complicating the issue is the fact that many devices do not have modular serviceability, that is, they are not structured in modular components easily removed and replaced by a non-technical user. Moreover, a single device may have different parts, each requiring a different maintenance schedule and maintenance procedure. Some parts may need earlier replacements or different cleaning techniques.

Spare parts

A hospital in a developing country attempting to acquire spare parts for a medical device that has broken down may face a number of hurdles. The spare parts may no longer be available, especially for medical devices that are approaching the end stages of their technical life. Because of lack of standardization, users may have difficulty finding the spare part that fits the exact medical device model that has broken down. Buying the part may require a credit card system (not yet a universal means of payment worldwide) and several months to arrive. Its cost may be prohibitive in relation to the importance given by health ministry officials to the usefulness of the device in question, or the hospital manager may decide that resources are better spent buying a new device than repairing a broken one. And the hospital may lack the required tools and expertise to install the part *(131)*.

Consumables

One of the most common problems confronting hospitals in low-resource countries is the lack of consumables. A consumable can only be used once or for a limited time and then needs to be discarded and replaced. Common examples are clinical laboratory test strips, electrocardiograph electrodes, electro-surgery tips, operating gowns, sterilizing liquids, dressings, reagents for diagnostic equipment, and radiography film. As with spare parts, lack of standardization can lead to fruitless searches for consumables that are compatible with a specific model of a specific medical device made by a specific manufacture. For low-resource countries, consumables can be a more difficult problem than spare parts or repair. Consumables incur an ongoing cost that is often not taken into account at the procurement stage. Some consumables may also require storage equipment, such as refrigeration, which may not be available.

5.2.2 Overcoming barriers to using medical devices

In many low-resource countries, under-use or misuse of devices is often linked to a lack of public funds and the consequent deficiencies of basic infrastructure. These problems will not disappear overnight. A possible solution to help lower the barriers to the use of medical devices would be to encourage countries to develop national health technology policies that include medical devices, and to integrate these policies—as most governments have done for pharmaceutical products—into their national health systems. Such policies, according to WHO, should aim at fostering equitable access to technology that is safe, effective, and of high quality, and that is used in a rational way *(2, 10)*.

Medical device design

There are several approaches to ensure that the design of a medical device fits the context in which the device is likely to be used.

One approach is human factors engineering, sometimes called ergonomics. Generally speaking, human factors engineering focuses on the device–user interface. This interface includes all components and accessories necessary to operate and maintain a device, such as controls, displays, software, operation, labels and instructions. Focusing on the user interface offers a unique opportunity to simplify the skills required to perform a procedure. And simplifying the operation of devices would enhance patient safety, whatever the resources of the country, but particularly for low-resource countries with few trained personnel.

However, the FDA cautions that simplicity does not always equate with safety, and even very simple devices can be dangerous. The following are FDA rules for an ergonomic medical device design, applicable to all settings *(161)*:

- make all facets of the design as consistent with user expectations as possible (i.e. intuitive rather than counter-intuitive);
- take into account the user's previous experience with medical devices and well-established conventions;
- design work stations, controls and displays around the basic capabilities of the user, such as strength, dexterity, memory, reach, vision, and hearing;
- design well-organized and uncluttered control and display arrangements; and
- ensure that the association between controls and displays is obvious, in order to facilitate proper identification and reduce the user's memory load.

For low-resource rural settings, attributes that manufacturers might consider for medical device design include: a robust reliability; ergonomic design; modular serviceability; procurability, i.e. a package containing relevant spare parts; repairability by local technicians; affordability; portability; power-sparing; and no or little disposable accessories.

A possible way forward for developing countries would include biomedical engineers being trained in developing countries, designing medical equipment for developing countries, and manufacturing the equipment in developing countries. Engineering design specifically conceived for developing countries can be envisioned for X-ray, ultrasound, electro-surgery, and clinical laboratory equipment, among other applications *(131)*.

Duke University, in the United States, is currently piloting a programme for training engineers in designing medical devices for developing countries. The main focus of the programme is on X-ray, ultrasound, electro-surgery and clinical laboratory equipment.[8]

Medical device management

An ideal medical device management approach for all countries should attempt to ensure that the medical device:

- complies with regulatory requirements;
- will be properly installed, maintained and calibrated by trained staff;
- will be used safely by a trained qualified operator;
- meets local human and environmental conditions; and
- is monitored by a post-market surveillance programme, which includes safety and adverse event reporting.

Incorporating these points into a medical device management system can be difficult and complicated, particularly due to human and financial limitations, but most of all because people are not aware of the importance of a good management system.

As previously mentioned, a robust management system can incorporate maintenance issues into its overall plan which may help overcome many maintenance problems.

Training

The lack of adequately trained health workers may be alleviated if countries develop a national human resources for health (HRH) plan. WHO is providing technical assistance for all countries to have a national HRH plan that deals with the training needs for all types of health workers, including those that will work with health technologies. This national HRH plan should be part of the overall national health policy and strategy, have an allocated budget, and be developed in consultation with all stakeholders.

The need for biomedical engineers (or similar country-specific positions) and training of health technology management professionals should be adequately considered during the development of the national HRH plan, also in consultation with the relevant stakeholders. The entities responsible at the country level with health technology management should also be actively involved in the development of this plan.

Having a central point person responsible for medical technologies within a health-care facility (similar to how a pharmacist is responsible for the distribution

---

8 http://www.ewh.org/index.php/programs/institutes/duke, accessed 13 July 2010.

and quality of pharmaceuticals) can be valuable. This role could be served by a trained biomedical engineer or another trained health technology management professional. This point person would ideally be knowledgeable on the technical specifications, installation procedures, and proper use of the technologies being used within a health-care facility, and be capable of training users in these health technologies. In addition, this health technology manager could provide assistance in the case of technological operative malfunctions, or assist with maintenance that may be needed. The position of health-care technology manager will vary from location to location, based on the financial resources of the health-care facility and in proportion to the number and types of health technologies being used. It may also be possible to have this role filled by a qualified contractor or consultant.

Any health-care providers engaged in using or maintaining medical devices should maintain and update their competencies regularly, as part of a continuous professional development plan *(162)*. If health technologies are used in home care, patients or their caregivers should be adequately trained to use the relevant technologies. Training and competence testing in the use of new medical devices could be valuable before the devices are put to use and could be a shared responsibility of the health-care provider and the manufacturer.

The lack of adequately trained health workers may also be alleviated if countries ensure that procurement contracts with manufacturers stipulate the provision of adequate training of staff in the use of procured devices during the technical life-cycle of the medical device. In addition, it may be valuable for country-specific regulatory authorities to mandate that instruction manuals for all imported medical devices be written in the language of the importing country, and require that medical device manufacturers make instruction manuals (including user and maintenance manuals) easily available and accessible.

5.3 Medical device innovation

Innovation is often intuitively perceived as a straightforward sequence of events. However, this view is too simplistic as there is rarely a single optimal solution to achieving a medical innovation *(90)*.

In addition, people decide whether or not to adopt an innovation based on various factors, such as its utility, its disruptive effect on existing habits, personal values, social status, and how keen individuals are to innovate *(163, 164)*. Within a defined population, there are several subpopulations with different abilities and willingness to adopt new technologies. These can be categorized as follows *(165)*.

- "innovators" constituting 2.5% of the population;
- "early adopters" constituting 13.5% of the population;
- "early majority" and "late majority", respectively constituting 34% each of the population;
- "laggards" constituting 16% of the population.

Therefore, when considering barriers to medical innovation, it is important to differentiate between obstacles to the innovation itself and obstacles to the uptake of medical innovation.

5.3.1 Barriers to innovation

Lack of funding and other support means that innovative ideas and innovative research may "die" at an intermediate stage of innovation between basic research and development. At this stage the risk for innovators is high and the likely profit uncertain. Private-sector investors tend to be wary of investing at this intermediate stage and prefer to fund more mature projects that are closer to commercialization. This intermediate stage is known as the "valley of death", where many good ideas and laboratory discoveries perish before having a chance to reach the market. (see Figure 5.3). To ease the safe passage of innovative ideas across the "valley of death", financial support from government or a non-profit agency is often required. *(166)*.

Health professionals often develop ideas for improving medical devices *(131)*. However, the main barrier they face is the difficulty of taking the innovative ideas through the design, testing, and manufacturing stages.

In low-resource settings, the origin of this barrier is lack of local research infrastructure and capacity to develop promising ideas. This is mainly due to lack of funds *(87)*. There is also little encouragement for

Figure 5.3 The "valley of death" for innovations

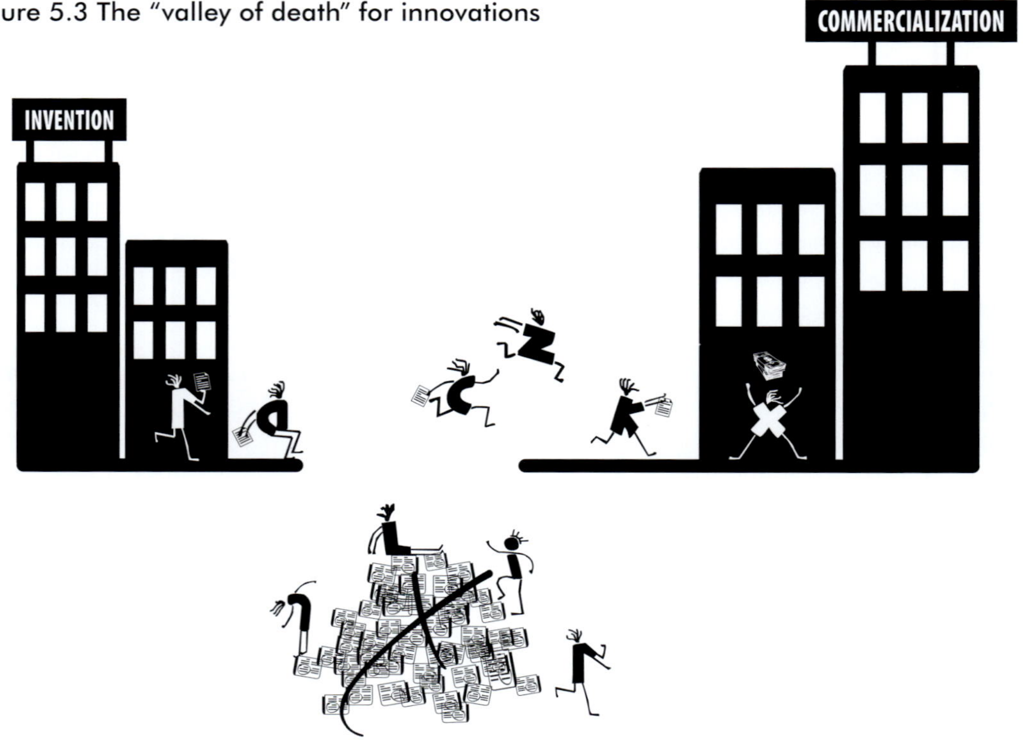

local innovation and few mechanisms for translating an innovative idea into a marketable product, even though local innovations may respond best to local needs *(167)*. Current innovation focuses on designing medical devices for low-resource settings by designers in high-resource settings: in other words, new ideas originate from those outside the context in which a device will be used.

Costs

Although regulatory requirements for the safety of medical devices perform an essential function, they impose an added financial burden on designers and manufacturers. This situation results in a dilemma: there is a need to encourage innovation and manufacturing of medical equipment in low-resource countries, and there is a need for all companies, including local companies in low-resource countries, to ensure that their products meet international safety standards. But to fulfil this condition, companies come up against the costs of regulation. However, regulation costs are not necessarily prohibitive and the public health perspective should have priority over industry interests.

Even technologies such as immunodiagnostic tests, which incur relatively low development costs, may become too costly for low-resource countries to produce if these costs are doubled or tripled when the products are submitted to the regulatory process required for licensing. Furthermore, the high costs of regulation can prompt companies to elude regulatory oversight, with the result that products of significant value to low-resource countries may not reach the market because they do not meet international safety standards *(5, 168)*.

As a practical example, internationally agreed upon standards require the batteries of portable defibrillators to be capable of functioning at temperatures as low as −10 °C. This standard might not be applicable to tropical settings, leaving manufacturers asking perplexing questions for which there are currently no answers. For example, should the same standards apply to the batteries of defibrillators to be used in tropical conditions? Can standards be adapted to local circumstances and conditions? Could lowering standards for batteries lead to lowering standards for other devices? What body could authorize such exceptions? Would medical device manufacturers who adhered to standards suffer a comparative disadvantage with respect to manufacturers who bend the rules? Could compliant manufacturers be permitted to market items at somehow lower levels of safety, quality, and/ or performance than are necessary for other devices?

Concerns surrounding these issues are currently hampering innovation of appropriate medical devices, particularly those for low-resource settings.

5.3.2 Barriers to appropriate innovation uptake

Resistance, reluctance, rejection

Obstacles to the introduction of any new method, procedure or piece of equipment exist in both industrialized and developing countries. Common barriers between high- and low-resource settings include reluctance to alter existing practices and lack of recognition of the need to train users and upgrade their skills *(155)*.

Even when it is clearly beneficial, the technology may be rejected simply because it is new and threatens existing practices *(87)*. Resistance can be based on reluctance of the medical community to adopt new technologies (*169, 170)*. Or, the new technology may be rejected by traditional communities proud of their own culture (*131, 171)*. The contrary—rejection of local brands in favour of international brands—is also found.

Inappropriate design

There is a difficult balance to strike between innovation that solves infrastructure problems and innovation that creates new needs. For instance, designing a device that uses disposable batteries may solve the problem of electricity shortage, but disposable batteries require a supply chain and waste management.

A specific example of an inappropriate design is the failure of affordable wooden-seat wheelchairs to achieve widespread use among people with disabilities in Nicaragua *(172)*. The simple wooden foldable seat was thought to be appropriate to local conditions—narrow doorways, high pavements and lack of access to buildings for wheelchair users. It was intended as a good replacement for existing hospital wheelchairs imported from high-resource settings that had hard tyres and non-removable armrests and footrests. However, the wooden chair required a cushion to prevent ulcer formation in people with spinal cord injuries. Although cushions were provided during the first year of use, most people in Nicaragua could not afford a replacement once the cushions wore out.

Cost of innovative devices

Most adopters of innovative technologies are caught between the desire to continually improve health and quality of life, and the need to limit health-care costs. Innovation is often associated with higher costs, although there are examples of new technology reducing the cost of diagnosis and treatment. Efforts to reduce costs inevitably mean that some promising innovations will diffuse, while others will not.

Conversely, high purchasing capacity and cost reimbursement arrangements can lead to inappropriate innovation uptake by stimulating the development of technologically-dominated health care, which in turn can lead to overuse of innovative, expensive devices that may not meet urgent clinical needs or benefit patients. An example is the frequent implantation of defibrillators in patients without clear evidence about which groups of patients would benefit most from the device and the procedure *(173)*. Another example concerns referrals for genetic tests, such as for the diagnosis of neurofibromatosis *(112)*.

5.3.3 Overcoming the barriers to medical innovation

Identifying local design priorities

The need and potential for identifying local design priorities is overwhelming. As discussed previously, medical devices developed in high-resource settings rarely function efficiently in low-resource settings. Therefore R&D in medical devices appropriate for the local context is urgently needed. There are some successful examples of how local innovation based on local design can be widely implemented, such as the Jaipur foot (Box 5.1).

Networking for innovation

Community local innovation networks could help with the free exchange of knowledge and experience from which imaginative ideas could emerge. Such networks could support innovation from proof of concept to proof of added value. Innovation institutes attached to universities, such as those at the University of Exeter Innovation Centre in the United Kingdom[9], the Innovation Center Denmark in Munich, Germany[10], the University of Cape Town Centre for Innovation and Entrepreneurship in South Africa,[11] and the Center for Integration of Medicine and Innovative Technology in the United States,[12] help to bridge the gap between academic research and commercial application.

The innovative health technologies initiative, launched by WHO in late 2009, invites manufacturers, institutions, universities, governments, individuals and non-profit organizations to submit information about innovative medical devices. The information can be in the form of existing concepts of technology or those that are still in development. The main criterion is that the innovations proposed have the potential to be appropriate for, accessible to, and affordable by low-resource countries.[13]

Partnerships for local innovation

Local innovation and development of medical devices is possible in settings where they are needed, provided that the infrastructure is available locally to:
- attract competent personnel;
- link invention and design to health-related needs;
- to use local materials and expertise; and
- launch the innovative product into appropriate networks for distribution to target populations.

Because local production of devices could increase their availability and contextual appropriateness, developing countries could explore new ways of building or strengthening innovation and development capacity. Through partnerships with medical device manufacturers in industrialized countries, developing countries can strengthen their own capacity to design and produce locally-appropriate medical devices. However, concerns about transparency, rule of law, business conduct and intellectual property will have to be addressed in order to encourage such partnerships *(176, 177)*.

A successful partnership for the design of appropriate medical devices should stimulate the creation of new ideas bearing on all stages of the medical device life-cycle, from concept to manufacture, marketing, and uptake. These new ideas should take into account local values and culture in order to avoid rejection. *(131)*

---

9   http://www.spaceforsuccess.co.uk/index.html (accessed 13 July 2010).
10 http://www.icdmuenchen.um.dk/en (accessed 13 July 2010).
11 http://www.gsb.uct.ac.za/gsbwebb/default.asp?intpagenr=559 (accessed 13 July 2010).
12 http://www.cimit.org (accessed 8 July 2010).
13 http://www.who.int/medical_devices/en/ (accessed 13 July 2010).

Box 5.2 Inexpensive innovation in action

A non-profit charitable trust and the manufacturing division of a hospital, located in the southern tip of India, have teamed up to manufacture high-quality intraocular lenses, suture needles, pharmaceuticals, surgical blades, and hearing aids for people in developing countries.[14] The products are used by eye-care institutions and ophthalmologists in more than 120 countries.

Founded in 1992 by a United States social entrepreneur, the company manufactures products that are affordable by people in developing countries. Intraocular lenses cost US$ 4–6 a piece, compared with the average price of US$ 100–150 in industrialized countries. Hearing aids sell for about US$ 50 a piece, versus around US$ 1500 in the United States . The price charged for a hearing aid is on a sliding scale: the poorest people pay nothing; the moderately poor pay a price that roughly covers the manufacturing costs (between US$ 20 and US$ 60); and for people who can afford to pay more, the price is greater than manufacturing costs to generate profit and offset losses on below-cost sales. In this way, sufficient revenue is gained for the company to be profitable and grow while serving the poorest people.

Source: (180).

Overcoming the cost barrier

The ways in which health care and its delivery are financed and the extent to which the use of innovative devices are reimbursed influence the rate at which medical innovations emerge and gain acceptance (178). For example, when coronary angioplasty was reimbursed at a level significantly greater than its cost, the procedure was widely adopted and continually improved technically (179), showing how adequate funding encourages continued investment in research and development and stimulates further innovation. In contrast, cochlear hearing implants were initially reimbursed at a rate that amounted to only a fraction of their cost. The result was to impair the uptake of this valuable, innovative, albeit expensive technology, and stall subsequent research and development which might have lowered the cost of the implants. These examples show how adequate funding encourages continued investment in research and development and stimulates further

innovation, and also how inadequate reimbursement can be a disincentive to innovation (179).

The cost barrier in developing countries could be partly overcome by the creation of locally-owned medical device companies manufacturing for local markets. Governments of some emerging economies subsidize research and development of medical equipment, particularly for the domestic production of X-ray, ultrasound machines, and patient monitoring devices for use in rural areas (87). It is likely that such companies will soon have the capability to design and produce medical equipment and supplies that will compete directly with products patented in Europe, Japan, and the United States. Box 5.2 provides an example of a successful inexpensive innovation.

5.4 Assistive devices

The need for assistive technology, especially in developing countries, is generally not fully known. There is little awareness of, and knowledge about, assistive technology in developing countries. Research has focused mainly on the design and production of mobility products, such as wheelchairs and lower-limb prostheses.

---

14   http://www.aravind.org/aurolab/index.asp (accessed 13 July 2010).

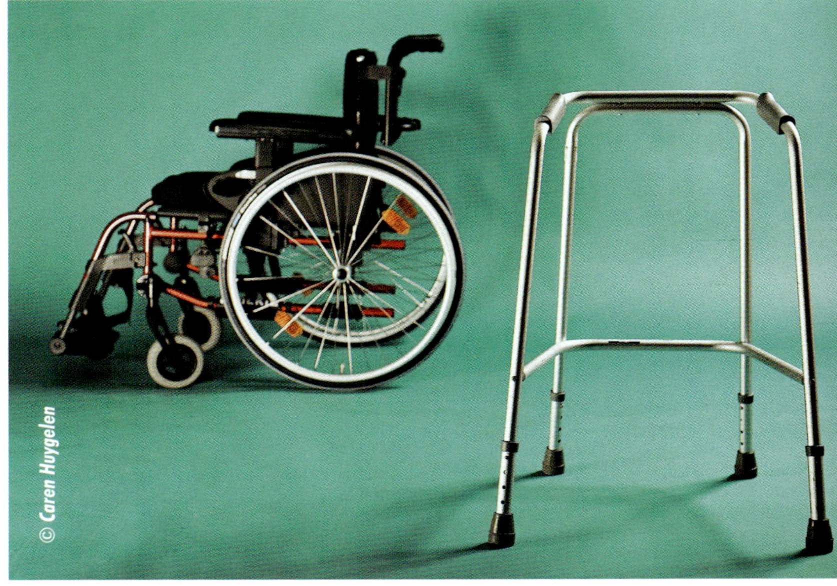

In many developing countries, only 5–15% *(96)* of people who require assistive devices and technologies have access to them. Reasons for this lack of access include inadequate production to meet global needs, the poor quality of some assistive devices, and prohibitive costs.

The development of a simple instrument to assess population needs for assistive devices and thereby allow for national planning would enable the development of policies to meet the needs of the growing number of people with disability and functioning problems. Ergonomic designs of assistive devices, such as wheelchairs and hand-driven tricycles, for use by people in developing countries should have a higher priority. In addition, development of new, efficient assistive devices, designed specifically for a given context and simple to use and produce with local resources, could help to substantially increase access to appropriate assistive devices.

5.5 Emerging themes

Table 5.3 lists the themes identified in this discussion related to the barriers and possible solutions to improve access to appropriate medical devices (that emerged from the country and specialist surveys, the expert focus groups and round table discussions, and the literature reviews). Each listed theme can be categorized into the crucial 4 components of the agenda to improve access to appropriate medical devices—Availability, Accessibility, Appropriateness, and Affordability. Lack of a regulatory framework is treated as an implicit issue in choosing and using medical devices and in medical device innovation.

5.5.1 Applying the 4 As to medical devices and medical interventions

It is possible to apply questions regarding Availability, Accessibility, Appropriateness, and Affordability to any of the key medical devices identified for the 15 global high-burden diseases. Applying such questions can lead to a possible research framework on the downstream factors associated with rationally choosing medical devices and effectively using them. As specific medical devices are not often considered in isolation, this approach can also be applied to complete medical interventions, such as the medical pathways involved in managing road traffic accidents (pages 69–75).

However, such an exercise is not an exact science. Rather, it could be used as a prompt to the areas that researchers, medical device choosers, and users should consider and apply to any of these key medical devices. After having performed a needs assessment according to the stepwise approach (see Section 3), the following 4 questions could be applied.
1. Is this medical device currently available?
2. Is it currently accessible?
3. Is it currently appropriate to the specific context?
4. is it affordable?

A negative answer to any of these questions requires further investigation that can be worked through to ascertain the main contributing factors to the negative answer. It is then possible to formulate a potential research framework for identifying clinical, technological, and/or process and systems knowledge-gaps to best improve access to appropriate medical devices and best address public health needs. Examples of how this exercise can be used and applied are shown below. The first focuses on oxygen equipment and the second on a complete road traffic accident intervention.

The answers to some of the 4 key questions may depend on local factors, but there are likely to be some common areas that can be more universally addressed, especially in low-income settings, such as the need for developing more appropriate designs, appropriate staff training programmes, and manageable maintenance systems.

Table 5.3 Summary of emerging themes relating to the barriers and possible solutions to access to appropriate medical devices

Theme	Barriers	Component(s) involved	Solutions	Components(s) involved
Choosing medical devices	Lack of information/biased information	Availability Accessibility Appropriateness Affordability	Improved information Rational decision-making	Appropriateness
	Fascination with technology	Appropriateness	Focus on public health needs	Appropriateness
	Deference to personal preference	Appropriateness	Focus on public health needs	Appropriateness
	Known and hidden costs	Affordability	Contain costs	Availability Accessibility Appropriateness Affordability
	Marketing practices	Availability Accessibility Appropriateness Affordability	Improve marketing practices	Availability Accessibility Appropriateness Affordability
	Lack of single nomenclature	Availability Accessibility Appropriateness	Develop a single system Rational decision-making	Appropriateness
	Shortcomings of clinical guidelines	Appropriateness	Improve clinical guidelines Rational decision-making	Appropriateness
Using medical devices	Inappropriate design	Appropriateness (affecting availability and accessibility)	Improve design	Appropriateness (leading to improved availability and accessibility)
	Context	Appropriateness (affecting availability and accessibility)	Improved design Partnerships for local innovation	Appropriateness (leading to improved availability and accessibility)
	Lack of appropriate management	Availability Accessibility	Improve management	Availability Accessibility Appropriateness Affordability
	Lack of appropriate staff training	Availability Accessibility	Improved staff training	Availability Accessibility
	Maintenance problems	Availability Accessibility Appropriateness Affordability	Improve medical device maintenance	Availability Accessibility Appropriateness Affordability
Innovation of medical devices	Lack of funding / infrastructure	Availability Accessibility Appropriateness Affordability	Increase funding and improved infrastructure Networking for innovation	Availability Accessibility Appropriateness Affordability
Uptake of medical devices	Resistance / Reluctance / Rejection	Availability Accessibility Appropriateness Affordability	Enhance appropriate designs Appropriate innovative solutions	Availability Accessibility Appropriateness Affordability
	Inappropriate design	Availability Accessibility Appropriateness Affordability	Identify local design priorities	Availability Accessibility Appropriateness Affordability
	Costs (including regulatory costs)	Availability Accessibility Appropriateness Affordability	Reduce costs	Availability Accessibility Appropriateness Affordability

Applying the "4A" questions: Oxygen equipment example

Question	Answer	Follow up
Is oxygen equipment (oxygen concentrators, cylinders, and pulse- oximeters) available?	Yes	Apply the 3 remaining key questions.
	No	Follow up with the question, Why not? Possible answers to the follow up question include: • There is no oxygen equipment at this health-care facility. • There is oxygen equipment but the oxygen cylinders are empty. • We have the oxygen cylinders and concentrators but we do not have any face masks and tubing to connect the oxygen left so cannot give oxygen. • There is oxygen equipment but we do not know how to use it. • There is oxygen equipment but not enough to meet the needs of our patients (the supply is very low).
Is oxygen equipment accessible?	Yes	Apply the 2 remaining key questions.
	No	Follow up with the question, Why not? Possible answers to the follow-up question include: • Only the hospital in town has oxygen equipment and there is no regular continuous oxygen supply, therefore we do not have any oxygen equipment in our local health centres or the emergency ambulances. • We have oxygen equipment but it is broken and we do not know how to fix it. • Health workers are not trained in the appropriate use of oxygen.
Is oxygen equipment appropriate?	Yes	Apply the final remaining key question.
	No	Follow up with the question, Why not? Possible answers to the follow-up question include: • The oxygen cylinders are too big and bulky and we have nowhere to put them. • We have the oxygen equipment but we do not know where to get the oxygen from when it runs out. • The oxygen equipment is suitable for use in our operating theatre but not for use in our paediatric ward (where it is needed for the treatment of pneumonia) and other surgical and obstetric wards, recovery room, intensive care unit and emergency room.
Is the oxygen equipment affordable?	Yes	Well done; (if all of the 4 key questions are answered positively) you have access to an appropriate, functioning medical devices system in place.
	No	Follow up with the question, Why not? Possible answers to the follow-up question include: • The oxygen equipment was donated but the running costs exceed the regular hospital supplies budget. • The cost of ensuring reliable oxygen supply systems is too much for us. • The cost of the oxygen equipment is manageable but we cannot afford to have an adequate supply of facemasks and tubing for every patient.

The answers given to the 4 key questions in this example highlight the main barriers to accessing appropriate oxygen equipment, including: hidden costs, maintenance problems, staff training issues, and inappropriate design for the specific context, in addition to the problem of overall lack of health funding and a weak health system.

Possible research areas derived from these answers include:
• Ascertaining the known and hidden costs of running and maintaining an adequate oxygen delivery system to give a more accurate reflection of total costs.
• Is there a need for a different design of oxygen equipment to make it more suitable to the local context in low-resource settings? If so, what would be the optimal design?
• What is the best and most cost-effective way of training all health staff in the use of oxygen equipment?
• Is there an easier and more manageable way in which oxygen equipment can be maintained? If so, what would be involved in this manageable maintenance system?

Example: Major road traffic accidents

The necessary emergency health system response to a road traffic accident can be illustrated in a series of diagrams. The following diagrams (taken from the Strengthening Emergency Care programme) highlight the overall system and outline the key equipment needed for the three main settings involved in emergency care—the ambulance, the accident unit (emergency room), and the operating theatre (183). A selected example of a medical device necessary for each setting illustrates how the "4 A" questions—availability, accessibility, appropriateness, and affordability—can be applied (as in the oxygen equipment example) to help identify necessary areas of future research. Ideally, this framework could be used for every medical device identified in each setting of emergency management. The selected examples are bag valve masks from the ambulance part of the process, blood transfusion equipment for the accident unit (emergency room), and an anaesthetic machine for the operating room.

OVERALL SYSTEM

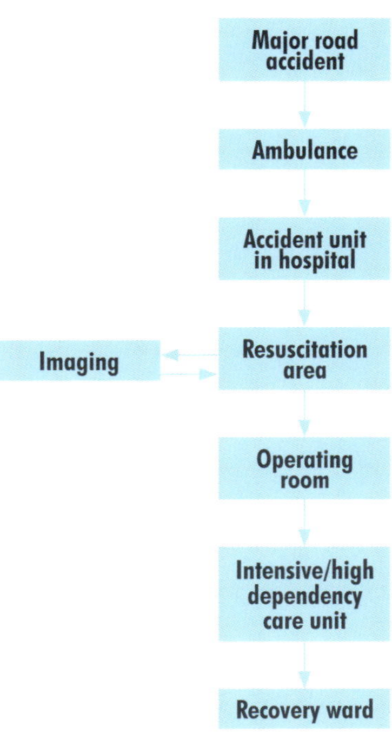

Reproduced with permission from the Strengthening Emergency Care programme — Advanced Life Support Group & Maternal Childhealth Advocacy.
http://www.mcai.org.uk/assets/content/documents/Introducing%20SEC%20to%20a%20new%20country.pdf

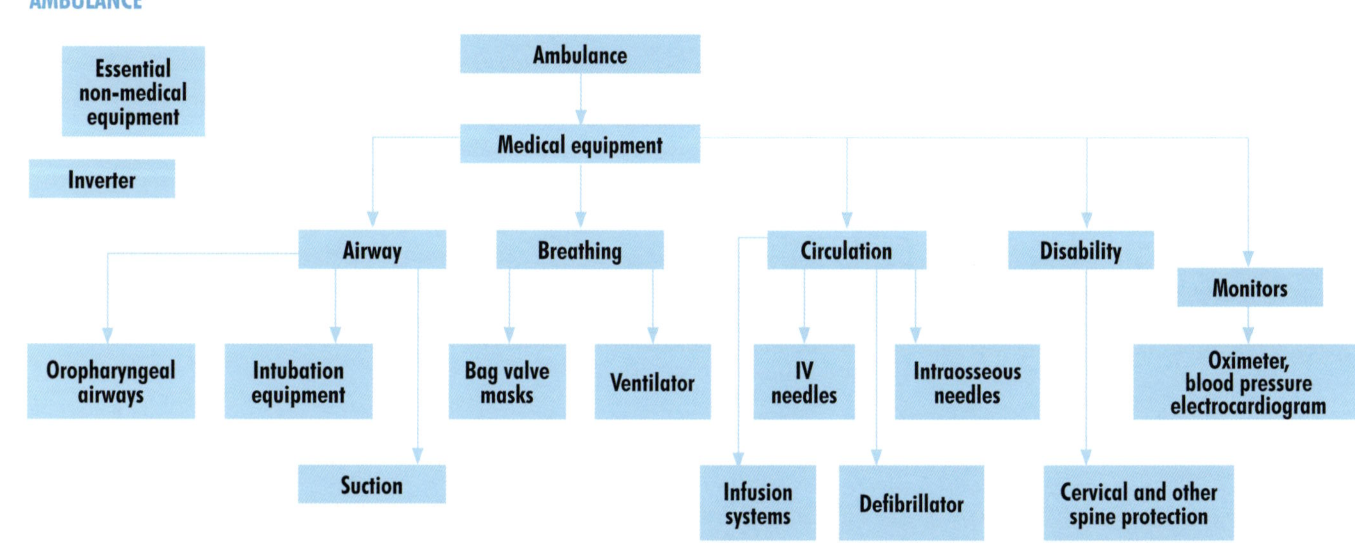

Reproduced with permission from the Strengthening Emergency Care programme — Advanced Life Support Group & Maternal Childhealth Advocacy.
http://www.mcai.org.uk/assets/content/documents/Introducing%20SEC%20to%20a%20new%20country.pdf

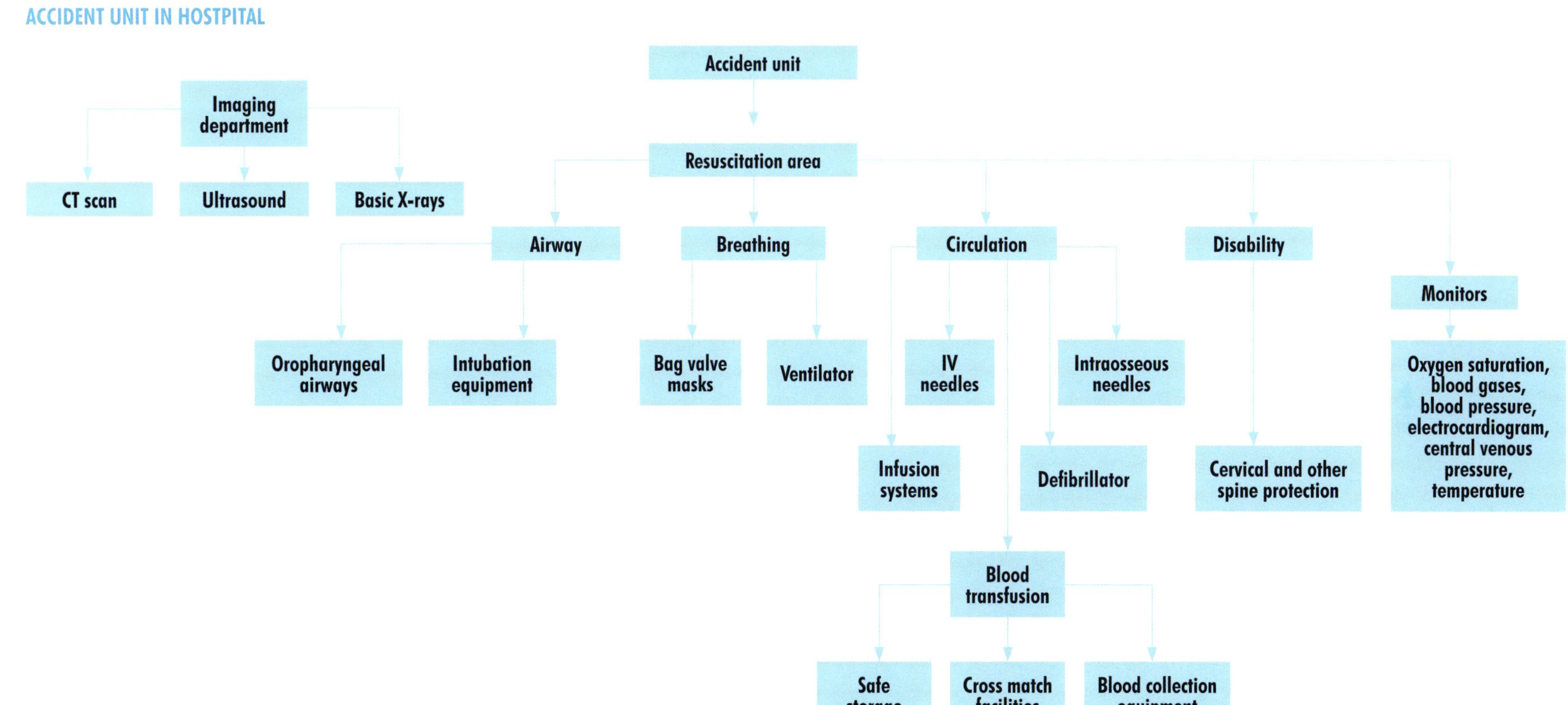

Reproduced with permission from the Strengthening Emergency Care programme — Advanced Life Support Group & Maternal Childhealth Advocacy.
http://www.mcai.org.uk/assets/content/documents/Introducing%20SEC%20to%20a%20new%20country.pdf

OPERATING THEATRE

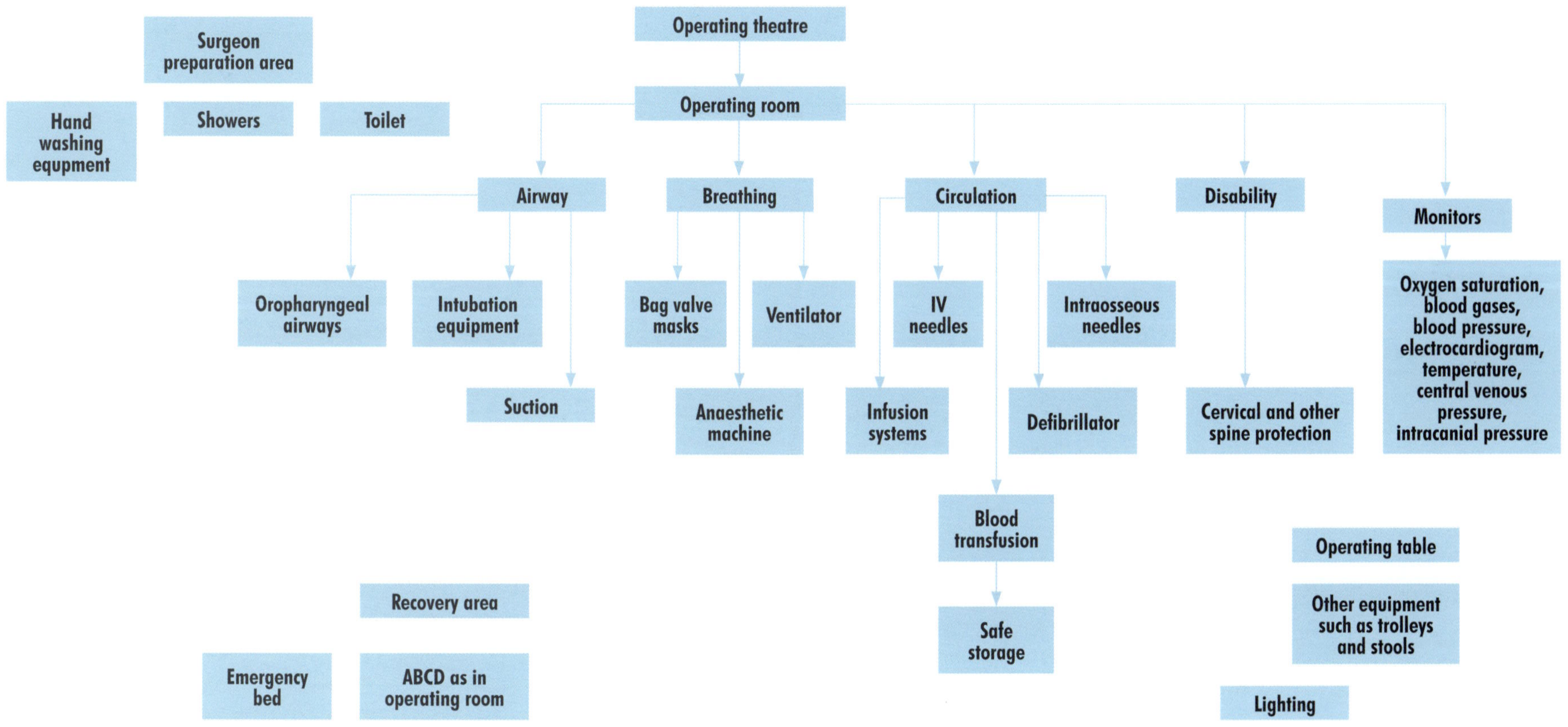

Reproduced with permission from the Strengthening Emergency Care programme — Advanced Life Support Group & Maternal Childhealth Advocacy.
http://www.mcai.org.uk/assets/content/documents/Introducing%20SEC%20to%20a%20new%20country.pdf

Applying the "4A" questions: example from the ambulance response

Question	Answer	Follow up
Are bag valve masks for inflating the lungs of a patient who is not breathing available?	Yes	Apply the 3 remaining key questions.
	No	Follow up with the question, Why not? Possible answers to the follow up question include: • There are no bag valve masks, either adult or paediatric, in the ambulance as no one realized their importance or they are taken away for use in the emergency rooms or wards. • There is only one bag valve mask available and it is too small for an adult (500ml for children aged up to one year, and 1800ml for older children and adults; both should be available).
Are bag valve masks accessible?	Yes	Apply the 2 remaining key questions.
	No	Follow up with the question, Why not? Possible answers to the follow-up question include: • There is only one ambulance man with the patient in the ambulance and no accompanying staff who can use the bag valve masks and accompanying health personnal is not trained. • There is a bag valve mask but it has a hole in it and cannot inflate the lungs and no one has reported this to the director of the health facility who needs to report to the regional health team responsible for equipment supply. • There are bag valve masks but the ambulance men do not know how to use them.
Are bag valve masks appropriate?	Yes	Apply the final remaining key question.
	No	Follow up with the question, Why not? Possible answers to the follow-up question include: • No one has thought that bag valve masks suitable for infants and older children and adults are essential in all ambulances. • The existing bag valve masks do not have an attached reservoir bag to ensure near 100% oxygen can be given when breathing for the patient.
Are bag valve masks affordable?	Yes	Well done; (if all of the 4 key questions are answered positively) you have access to an appropriate, functioning medical devices system in place.
	No	Follow up with the question, Why not? Possible answers to the follow-up question include: • Originally bag valve masks were donated but they became damaged and the regional health team did not have funds to replace them. • The cost of ensuring constantly-working bag valve masks is too much for us (extremely unlikely, since the device is very inexpensive). • The cost of bag valve masks is manageable but we cannot afford to dispose this as one is supposed to use a new set on every patient (as requested by our infection control department).

The answers given to the 4 key questions in this example highlight the main barriers to accessing appropriate bag valve masks to breathe for patients who have stopped breathing (a common emergency) including: maintenance problems, staff training issues, inappropriate design for the specific context, in addition to the problem of overall lack of health funding and a weak health system.

Possible research areas derived from these answers include:
• Ascertaining the known and hidden costs of running and maintaining bag valve masks to give a more accurate reflection of total costs.
• Discussions with infection control to find a solution so that bag valve masks can be safely cleaned between patient use.
• What is the best and most cost-effective way of training all health staff in the use of bag valve masks?
• Can the system afford a paramedic to accompany the driver of the ambulance so that resuscitation can continue during the journey.

Applying the "4A" questions: example from the accident unit: blood transfusion equipment

Question	Answer	Follow up
Is blood transfusion equipment (e.g. laboratory group and cross-match facilities and equipment, storage bags, and a storage refrigerator) available?	Yes	Apply the 3 remaining key questions.
	No	Follow up with the question, Why not? Possible answers to the follow up question include: • There is no blood transfusion equipment at this health-care facility. • There is blood transfusion equipment but only for cross-match and immediate transfusion: there is no storage refrigerator. • There is blood transfusion equipment but there is nobody in the laboratory who knows how to use it. • There is blood transfusion equipment but staff is on duty only during the morning shift from Monday to Friday. • There is blood transfusion equipment but not enough to meet the needs of our patients. • There is a blood transfusion storage refrigerator but it has broken down and we do not have a technician to repair it.
Is blood transfusion equipment accessible?	Yes	Apply the 2 remaining key questions.
	No	Follow up with the question, Why not? Possible answers to the follow-up question include: • Only one hospital in the region has blood transfusion equipment and it is too far away from our facility to access in an emergency. • We have blood transfusion equipment but there are too few trained staff available to check safely that the blood has been correctly cross-matched and safely stored before use.
Is blood transfusion equipment appropriate?	Yes	Apply the final remaining key question.
	No	Follow up with the question, Why not? Possible answers to the follow-up question include: • The blood storage refrigerator relies on electricity, which is frequently not available for many hours at a time and therefore we cannot safely store blood in it. • We have the blood transfusion equipment but we do not know where to get more replacement reagents and blood storage bags when they run out.
Is the blood transfusion equipment affordable?	Yes	Well done; (if all of the 4 key questions are answered positively) you have access to an appropriate, functioning medical devices system in place.
	No	Follow up with the question, Why not? Possible answers to the follow-up question include: • The blood transfusion refrigerator is too expensive for our health-care system. • The blood transfusion refrigerator was donated, but the running costs are too expensive for us to afford. When there is no electricity we have to use a generator, which is prohibitively expensive on fuel or there is no fuel available. • The cost of the blood transfusion equipment is manageable but we cannot afford to replenish consumables for the laboratory. • We cannot afford to pay a laboratory technician to be available 24 hours a day.

Possible research areas derived from these answers include:
• Developing a blood storage system that will work reliably when the mains electricity fails in low-resource settings.
• What is the best and most cost-effective way of training all health staff in the use of blood transfusion equipment?
• Is there an easier and more manageable way in which blood transfusion equipment can be maintained? If so, what would be involved in this manageable maintenance system?

Applying the "4A" questions: example from the operating room: anaesthetic machine

Question	Answer	Follow up
Is an anaesthetic machine available?	Yes	Apply the 3 remaining key questions.
	No	Follow up with the question, Why not? Possible answers to the follow up question include: • There is no oxygen available at this health-care facility, and oxygen is needed for the anaesthetic machine to function safely. • There is an anaesthetic machine but the oxygen cylinders needed to supply it are empty. • We have an anaesthetic machine but no anaesthetic agents to use in it. • There is an anaesthetic machine but there are no trained anaesthetists available to use it. • There is one anaesthetic machine but often there is a need to undertake more than one operation at a time and therefore more than one is needed.
Is an anaesthetic machine accessible?	Yes	Apply the 2 remaining key questions.
	No	Follow up with the question, Why not? Possible answers to the follow-up question include: • Only the regional hospital has an anaesthetic machine. We do not have any anaesthetic machines at our local health centres and yet we are required to undertake urgent surgery (currently we use ketamine by IV infusion). • We have an anaesthetic machine but it is broken or unsafe and we do not know how to fix it: there is no biomedical support available. • We have too few anaesthetists on staff; we can only use the anaesthetic machine when they are on duty.
Is an anaesthetic machine appropriate?	Yes	Apply the final remaining key question.
	No	Follow up with the question, Why not? Possible answers to the follow-up question include: • The anaesthetic machine is too complicated for our untrained anaesthesia provider and therefore unsafe • We have an anaesthetic machine but we do not know where to get more anaesthetic agents when they run out. • Frequently the electricity in our facility is not available. Our anaesthetic machine relies on electricity to function. There is no manual back up or other way of using the machine when the electricity fails.
Is an anaesthetic machine affordable?	Yes	Well done; (if all of the 4 key questions are answered positively) you have access to an appropriate, functioning medical devices system in place.
	No	Follow up with the question, Why not? Possible answers to the follow-up question include: • The anaesthetic machine was donated but the running costs are too expensive for us to afford, especially the costs of the anaesthetic agents and the annual servicing. • There is no funding allotted to train anaesthetists or train non-physician health worker to deliver anaesthesia. • This anaesthetic machine requires an appropriately trained doctor to use it and we do not have enough doctors locally.

The answers given to the 4 key questions in this example highlight the main problems to accessing appropriate oxygen equipment including: hidden costs, maintenance problems, staff training issues, and inappropriate design for the specific context, in addition to the problem of overall lack of health funding and a weak health system.

Possible research areas derived from these answers include *(182)*:
• Ascertaining the known and hidden costs of running and maintaining the anaesthetic machine to give a more accurate reflection of total costs
• Is there a need for a different design of an anaesthetic machine to make it more suitable to the local context in low-resource settings? If so, what would be the optimal design? In fact, low-cost alternative anaesthetic machines could be researched for this facility.
• What is the best and most cost-effective way of training our health personnel to provide anaesthesia?
• Is there an easier and more manageable way in which the anaesthetic machine can be serviced and maintained? If so, what would be involved in this manageable maintenance system?
• Are there alternative volatile agents that can be used in the existing anaesthetic machine that could be more affordable?

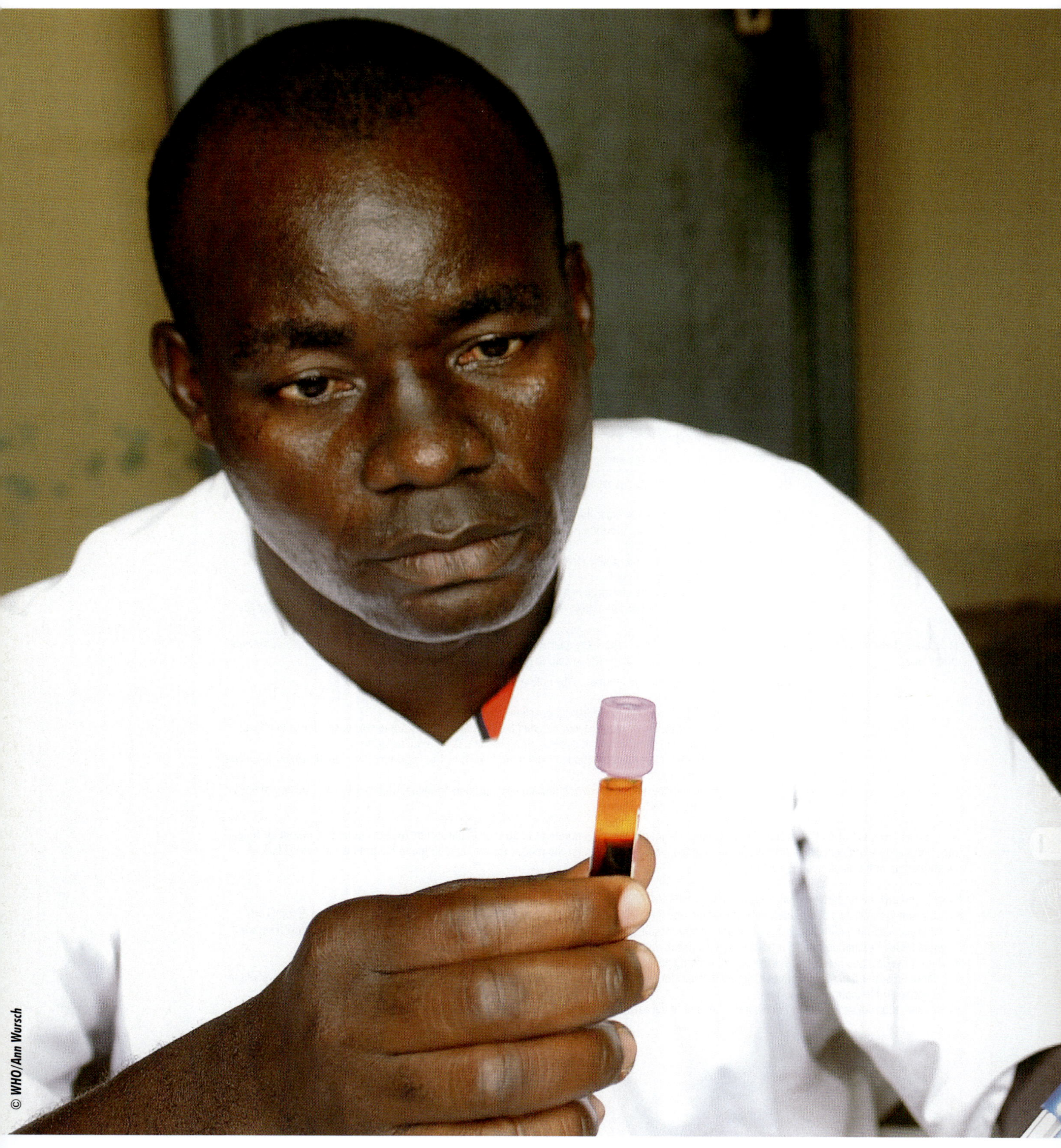

Towards appropriate medical devices: options for future research

6

The final section of the report brings together all the information and findings in the preceding sections. It suggests how applying the crucial 4 components—Availability, Accessibility, Appropriateness, and Affordability—to current and future high-burden diseases and risk factors as well as some cross-cutting issues associated with them (e.g. injection safety, study design, laboratory diagnostic tools) may help improve access to appropriate medical devices. The results of this exercise suggest several areas of research that could be taken forward.

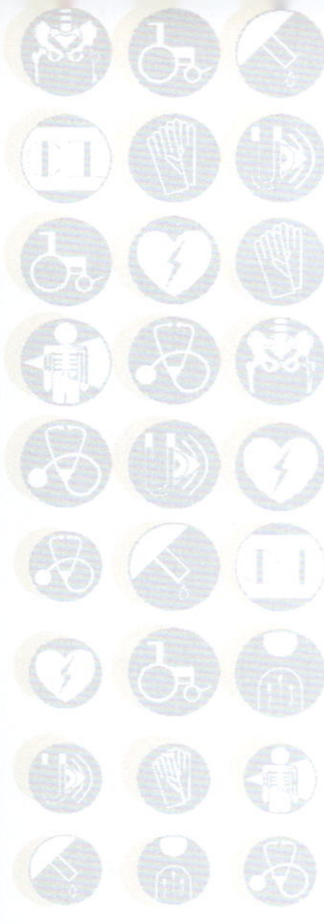

6.1 Methodology

In order to help inform any potential research agenda in access to appropriate medical devices, the *PMD* project conducted a scoping search of the literature on recent or current research in the field of medical devices. This scoping search could be the basis of a future systematic literature review.

The scoping search aimed to identify studies in the "pipeline" and to discover which medical devices are currently of scientific and developmental interest. Consistent with the overall methodology of this report, the scoping search was based on terms related to high-burden diseases and some cross-cutting themes. We used Ovid Medline as the main medical database. Please see http://www.who.int/medical_devices/access/en/index.html for the full search strategy.

To verify the findings from the scoping search, we identified and asked clinical specialists from each of the 15 high-burden diseases to comment on our analysis. We then drafted some possible areas of future research in each disease option which were reviewed by a second specialist. These research areas are couched in terms of medical device availability, accessibility, appropriateness, and affordability.

There are several limitations associated with this methodology.

- Using global burden of disease estimates as an indication of public health needs for medical devices produces research priorities pertinent more to global than to regional or national priorities.
- As ongoing research is included in the scoping exercise, there is no evidence yet that the results of this research will bring therapeutic benefits.
- Using management of specific diseases as a starting point for determining future research needs excludes research needed on medical devices for general use, such as hospital beds, sterilizers, and operating lamps.
- The proposed research areas represent the result of a highly selective process and therefore do not cover all possible relevant research areas.
- Assessing the need for research in specific areas calls for knowledge about current ongoing research. Yet, in the notoriously competitive environment of medical device development, information about their R&D is rarely publicly available.
- A constraining factor in the preparation of the suggested research agenda has been the paucity in the clinical guidelines consulted, of specific medical devices required for recommended health-care pathways.
- Research on tools for the prevention of ill-health and disability is a vital need but beyond the scope of the suggested research agenda.

However, the following findings could be used as a potential basis to form a more robust and comprehensive research agenda in the future.

6.2 Results

6.2.1 Scoping exercise

Past meta analyses of clinical trials using medical devices for cardiovascular disease, TB, and diabetes were searched in the Cochrane database. This search indicated that less than 10 meta analyses have been completed for TB and less than 10 for diabetes. For cardiovascular disease almost 200 meta analyses on therapeutic medical devices have been published. According to the scoping search, the three conditions which currently attract the most research in medical devices are cancer, HIV/AIDS, and perinatal conditions. However, for the majority of global high-burden diseases, there is currently very limited research under way in medical devices. Please see http://www.who.int/medical_devices/access/en/index.html for the tabulated results of the scoping exercise.

6.3 Future research areas in cross-cutting areas

There are numerous cross-cutting themes in the high-burden diseases that relate to medical devices. Four of the topics—study design and clinical outcome, laboratory diagnostic tools, labour-saving devices, and injection safety—have been selected for the examples below.

6.3.1 Study design and clinical outcome

An area of research that is of particular relevance to clinicians and health decision-makers is information about relevant clinical outcomes. The key question which needs to be answered is: what information is needed for clinicians and health decision-makers to make a fully informed decision on a medical technology, no matter whether it is an in vitro diagnostic or another area of medical device technology? Currently, study design for market approval is focused on compliance with regulatory requirements, which include the safety and effectiveness of the medical device. To know the benefit of a new medical technology compared to existing technologies, comparative studies with relevant patient outcomes need to be performed. To date, most research on new technologies has not provided this essential information. Therefore, development of improved study designs appropriate for technologies and medical devices, which include relevant patient outcomes, is necessary.

Bibliography

Sedrakyan A. et al., A framework for evidence evaluation and methodological issues in implantable device studies. *Medical Care*, 2010, 48(6 Suppl):S121–8.

Burns LR. et al. Assessment of medical devices: How to conduct comparative technology evaluations of product performance. *International Journal of Technology Assessment in Health Care*, 2007, 23(4):455–463.

Horvath AR. Grading quality of evidence and strength of recommendations for diagnostic tests and strategies. *Clinical Chemistry, 2009*, 55(5):853–855.

6.3.2 Laboratory diagnostic tools

The universal lack of standardization in the medical device arena (such as the lack of standardized laboratory equipment and consumables) has great impact on diagnostic tools and negatively affects their effective use. Solutions to allow for greater standardization would be most beneficial and help to encourage universal use of "generic" diagnostic tools, which in turn could lead to standardized procurement practices, which has many potential advantages. As already mentioned in this report, this concept could apply to medical devices in general, not just diagnostics. "Generic", "compatible", "standarized", and "interoperable" equipment could lower costs, make training more efficient, make consumables easier to find, and facilitate the creation of generic technical specifications for procurement.

Availability and accessibility

One of the most common problems in low-resource countries is the lack of consumables, some of which can only be used once or for a limited time before they need to be discarded and replaced. Recurrent costs, such as renewing reagents for diagnostic kits and staff training, can amount to more than 80% of the total cost of a device *(130, 131)*.

Point-of-care diagnostic testing, which brings laboratory diagnostic technology to the patient, can allow for monitoring at home or at the primary health-care level. Such testing is growing in popularity, in high- and low-resource settings, particularly where patients would otherwise have to travel long distances to reach a health facility with a well-equipped laboratory. Good quality, easy-to-use point-of-care HIV test kits have been developed but are generally lacking for other infectious diseases because market incentives have been lacking. Development of simple, affordable test kits for other high-burden diseases would be useful in meeting public health needs. Such tests would be most useful if they require no electricity, refrigeration or access to clean water, and are easy to use with little or no training.

Appropriateness and affordability

In some diseases, such as malaria, treatment is cheaper than the diagnostic test. Over-treatment is therefore a problem, especially if this can lead to drug resistance (see the chapter on malaria below). Development of affordable, robust in vitro diagnostic tests based on microchip technology that allows for highly sensitive diagnoses of several diseases concurrently may help to solve the problem of over-treatment.

Development of simple, affordable, and reliable sensitivity tests for bacterial and viral antigens could replace culture systems to detect the presence of pathogens. This development could result in many high-burden infections being diagnosed more effectively and efficiently.

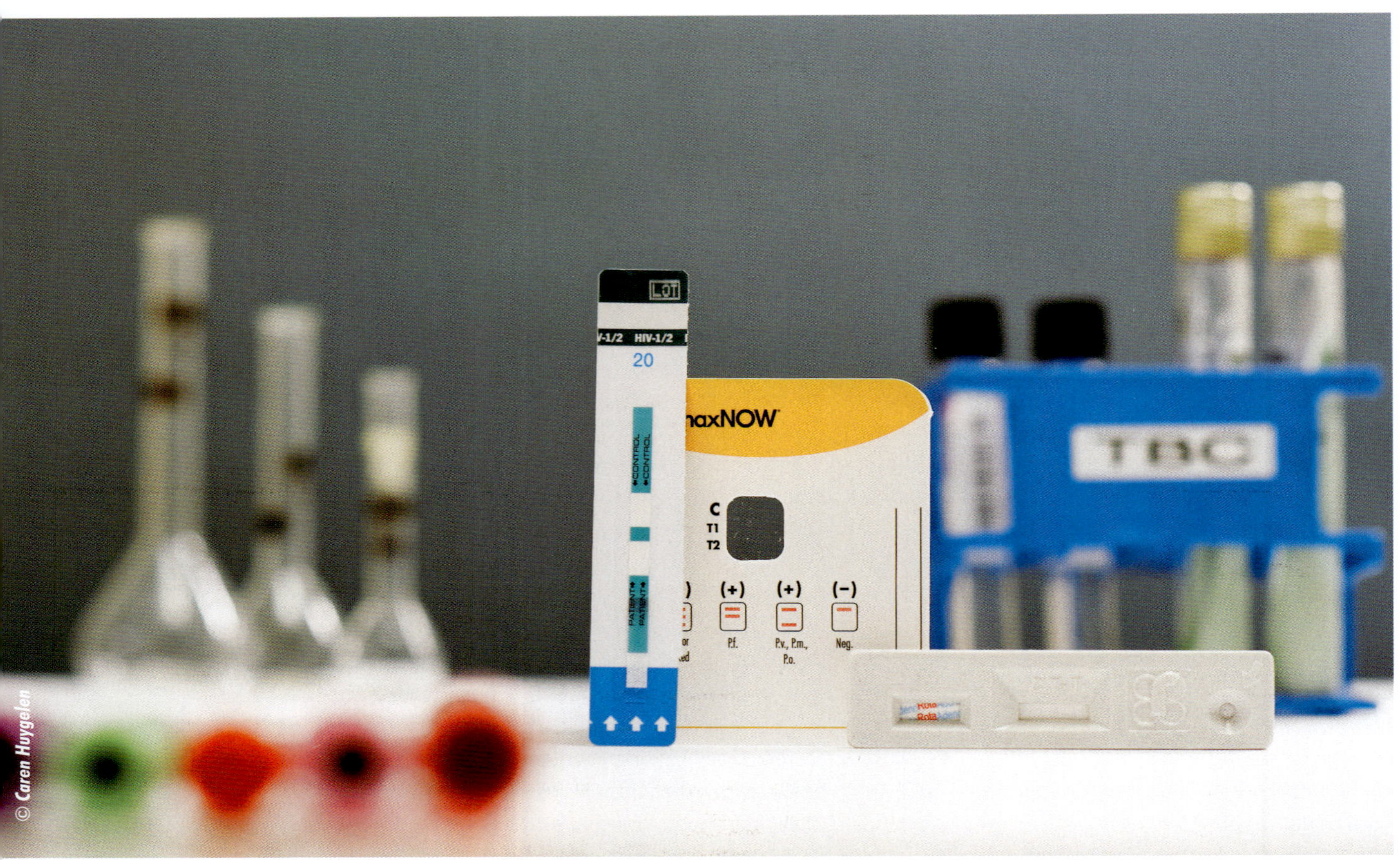

Neglected tropical diseases

Lack of diagnostic techniques is a particular issue for neglected tropical diseases, and these diseases deserve a special mention here.

WHO currently lists 17 neglected tropical diseases (NTDs)—neglected in the sense they do not have high visibility on the international health scene. Such diseases are concentrated almost exclusively in impoverished populations: more than 70% of affected countries are low-income or lower middle-income economies. The NTDs are mostly infectious diseases caused by bacteria, viruses or parasites that thrive in tropical places with unsafe water, poor sanitation, and limited access to basic health care. The six most common NTDs are schistosomiasis (200 million people infected), lymphatic filariasis (120 million), blinding trachoma (80 million), onchocerciasis (37 million), Chagas disease (13 million), and leishmaniasis (12 million). There is considerable social stigma attached to each of these diseases.

People in remote areas often become ill or die before their disease is diagnosed. Diagnosing at an early stage of the infection is a common need for most NTDs. Industry incentive to develop new diagnostic tools is low for a market unlikely to produce a reasonable return on investment. However, development of these diagnostic tools could be in the interests of industry if they could be procured by UN organizations or donating agencies, therefore guaranteeing industry a predefined market. Whatever the funding mechanism, the development of rapid, portable, and affordable diagnostic tools that are easy to use in a field setting is urgently required for many of these NTDs and consequently, would benefit many of the most underprivileged people and populations in the world.

Cutting-edge technologies

In both high- and low-resource settings, automated health-care technologies could allow fewer skilled technicians to operate a larger volume of diagnostic laboratory test equipment, thereby saving human resource costs. Development of a universally accepted standardized automated laboratory testing system may help to achieve this possibility.

Bibliography

Foundation for Innovative New Diagnostics. FIND, 2009 (http://www.finddiagnostics.org/, accessed 27 February 2010).

Boelaert M et *al. Evaluation of rapid diagnostic tests: visceral leishmaniasis. Nature Reviews Microbiology*, 2007, S30–S39.

Control of neglected tropical diseases. Geneva, World Health Organization, 2010 (http://www.who.int/neglected_diseases/en/, accessed 27 February 2010).

Esterre P et al. The impact of 34 years of massive DEC chemotherapy on Wuchereria bancrofti infection and transmission: the Maupiti cohort. *Tropical Medicine and International Health,* 2001, 6(3):190–195.

Kaplan W, Laing R. *Priority medicines for Europe and the world.* Geneva, World Health Organization, 2004 (WHO/EDM/PAR/2004.7).

Macroeconomics and health: investing in health for economic development. Report of the Commission on Macroeconomics and Health. Geneva, World Health Organization, 2001.

Melrose WD, Durrheim DD, Burgess GW. Update on immunological tests for lymphatic filariasis. *Trends in Parasitology,* 2004, 20(6):255–257.

Otani MM et al. WHO comparative evaluation of serologic assays for Chagas disease. *Transfusion,* 2009, 49(6);1076–1082.

6.3.3 Telemedicine and labour-saving technologies

Telemedicine is most used where there is a lack of specialized health personnel (e.g. in low-income settings, where health worker shortage is a serious, chronic problem). Telemedicine and labour-saving technologies could have a large potential to benefit patients in low-income settings. However, nothing can replace the need for a vast increase in the number of health workers in low-income settings. In high-income settings, labour-saving technologies could help health workers who are currently struggling to meet the needs of a growing elderly population.

Availability and accessibility

Research on labour-saving devices is currently mostly aimed at high-income countries, rendering the areas of research to be mostly high-tech.

Technology, such as remote patient monitoring, videoconferencing, telemedicine (including telediagnostics, telehealth, eHealth, and point-of-care systems) is allowing more patients to receive care outside the hospital setting and more health-care providers to offer their services without spending valuable time travelling to patients' homes (a particularly valuable labour-saving advantage for providers in remote areas).

Remote home-care technologies are being advocated as a means of reducing a patient's dependency on health-care personnel. However, it is necessary to perform economic analyses to verify the extent to which a specific technology results in a substantial lowering of demand on a health-care system.

Remote communications systems, such as interactive remote videoconferencing, or teletraining, telediagnostics and a host of other Web-based technologies, can be used in low- and high-income countries. Such technologies can cut costs in time, effort and money needed to train health professionals. Home telehealth is assumed to be cost saving from the perspective of the health-care system and insurance provider. Again, further rigorous research is needed to confirm if this assumption is true or not. Telerobotic surgery is an application of telemedicine that is currently used only in high-resource countries, but its cost-effectiveness has yet to be evaluated.

Current evidence suggests that home telehealth technology has the potential to reduce costs, but its impact from societal, social, and psychological perspectives remains uncertain. Therefore, further research is needed regarding ethical concerns, policies, reimbursement and legal implications.

Appropriateness and affordability

Labour-saving technology can also refer to assistive products. Identification of the types of assistive technologies that enable people to exercise their human rights, including maximizing opportunities to study and earn a living would be beneficial. Ways of enhancing access to assistive products and appropriately redesigning home environments need further development, in both low- and high-income settings.

Bibliography

Agree EM, Freedman VA, Sengupta M. Factors influencing the use of mobility technology in community-based long-term care. *Journal of Aging & Health*, 2004, 16(2):267–307.

Alverson DC et al. One size doesn't fit all: bringing telehealth services to special populations. *Telemedicine Journal & E-Health*, 2008, 14(9):957–963.

Anvari M. Remote telepresence surgery: the Canadian experience. *Surgical Endoscopy*, 2007, 21(4):537–541.

Charness N. Bosman EA. Age-related changes in perceptual and psychomotor performance: implications for engineering design. *Experimental Aging Research*, 1994, 20(1):45–59.

Chetney R. Home care technology and telehealth— the future is here. *Home Healthcare Nurse*, 2003, 21(10):645–646.

Cook A et al. Prospective evaluation of remote, interactive videoconferencing to enhance urology resident education: The Genitourinary Teleteaching Initiative. *The Journal of Urology*, 2005, 174 (5):1958–1960.

Haselkorn A. The future of remote health services: summary of an expert panel discussion. *Telemedicine Journal & E-Health*, 2007, 13(3):341–347.

Kelly D, McLoone S, Dishongh T. Enabling affordable and efficiently deployed location based smart home systems. *Technology & Health Care*, 2009, 17(3):221–235.

King G, Farmer J. What older people want: evidence from a study of remote Scottish communities. *Rural & Remote Health*, 2009, 9(2):1166.

Metaxiotis K, Ptochos D, Psarras J. E-health in the new millennium: a research and practice agenda. *International Journal of Electronic Healthcare*, 2004, 1(2):165–175.

Van Oost RM et al. Introduction of assistive devices: home nurses' practices and beliefs. *Journal of Advanced Nursing,* 2006, 54(2):180–188.

Polisena J et al. Home telehealth for chronic disease management: a systematic review and an analysis of economic evaluations. *International Journal of Technology Assessment in Health Care*, 2009, 25(3):339–349.

Scott RE, Ndumbe P, Wootton R. An e-health needs assessment of medical residents in Cameroon. *Journal of Telemedicine & Telecare*, 2005, 11(Suppl 2):S78–80.

Tsiachristas et al. *Medical innovations and labor savings in health care: An exploratory study.* The Hague, Aarts De Jong Wilms Goudriaan Public Economics bv (APE) and Maastricht University, 2009.

Eadie LH, Seifalian AM, Davidson BR. Telemedicine in surgery. *British Journal of Surgery,* 2003, 647–658.

Bergmo TS. Can economic evaluation in telemedicine be trusted? A systematic review of the literature. *Cost Effectiveness and Resource Allocation* 2009, 7:18 (http://www.resource-allocation.com/content/7/1/18, accessed 8 July 2010).

Johnston K et al. The cost-effectiveness of technology transfer using telemedicine. *Health policy planning*, 19(5):302–309.

6.3.4 Safe injections

Syringes and needles are among the most commonly used medical devices in the world. In 2000, WHO estimated that every year in developing countries, 16 billion injections are given, among which almost 40% were given with reused, unsterilized injection equipment. Based on this evidence, WHO

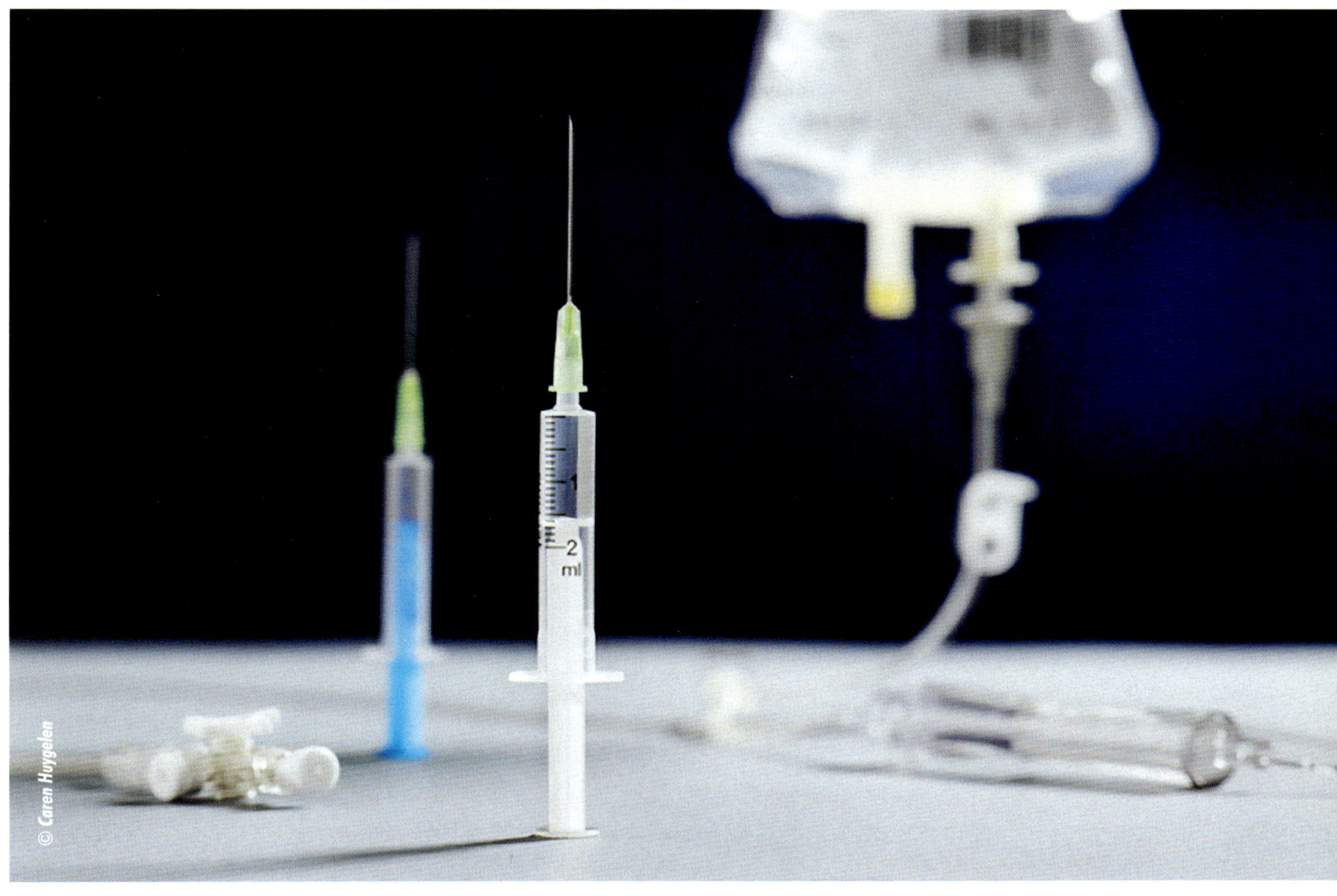

established a programme to promote the rational and safe use of injections worldwide. WHO has defined a safe injection as one that does not harm the recipient, does not expose the provider to any avoidable risk, and does not result in any waste that is dangerous to other people. Long-term improvements of injection practices may be possible through prevention: through training, raising awareness, and continuous provision of sufficient quantities of good-quality injection devices.

Reuse and needle stick injury prevention injection devices: availability and accessibility

Disposable single-use syringes were devised in order to reduce the risk of a contaminated needle infecting a subsequent patient or vaccine recipient. However, in actual practice, disposable syringes are often used more than once, particularly in low-resource areas. People in low-income settings also incur the risk of needle-stick injuries through inappropriate waste management systems. Development of efficiently managed waste disposable systems may help to greatly reduce this risk.

Engineered syringes that prevent reuse and needle-stick injuries are much safer than traditional syringes. However, they are more expensive and often unaffordable in low-resource countries. Development of syringes that prevent reuse and needle-stick injuries but are designed and manufactured to make them more affordable to low-resource countries could potentially decrease the preventable harms to patients and health-care workers.

Biodegradable needles have been used on a limited scale. Development of single-use biodegradable needles that require no waste disposal systems could help to eliminate the risk of cross-contamination and needle-stick injuries.

Another innovative option to prevent unsafe injection practices is the development of needle-free technologies. Further development of needle-less injection devices for transdermal administration, such as jet injectors, patches and transmucosal sprays, could potentially help to solve most of the risks associated with needle use.

Bibliography

Hirschberg HJHB et al. Bioneedles™ as vaccine carriers. *Vaccine*, 2008, 26:2389–2397.

Hutin Y et al. Best infection control practices for intradermal, subcutaneous, and intramuscular needle injections. *Bulletin of the World Health Organization*, 2003, 81:491–500.

Landscape analysis: trends in vaccine availability and novel vaccine delivery technologies: 2008–2025. PATH/World Health Organization, 2009.

Hauri AM, Armstrong GL, Hutin YFD. The global burden of disease attributable to contaminated injections given in health care settings. *International Journal of STD & AIDS,* 2004, 15:7–16.

WHO best practices for injections and related procedures toolkit. Geneva, World Health Organization, 2010, http://whqlibdoc.who.int/publications/2010/9789241599252_eng.pdf.

6.4 Future research areas in global high-burden diseases

A selection of the current and future high-burden diseases is listed and discussed below. The current high-burden diseases are discussed before the future trends in high-burden diseases. The focus is mostly on the research areas required in low-income settings, as access to appropriate medical devices is severely lacking in these areas. However, where appropriate, cutting-edge technologies for both high- and low-income settings are also mentioned as a potential future research area. As mentioned in the limitations (see Chapter 6.1), it is important to note that as the scoping exercise focused on ongoing research in high-burden diseases, there is currently limited evidence that the results of this research will bring therapeutic benefits.

The context of each disease is summarized before highlighting some of the possible future research required to help enhance the agenda to improve access to appropriate medical devices by increasing medical device availability, accessibility, appropriateness, and affordability.

6.4.1 Perinatal conditions

An estimated 3.3 million babies are stillborn every year—babies who do not breathe at birth are often classed as stillborn even though some of them could be successfully resuscitated if appropriate equipment and staff training were available. Every year, 4 million infants die within 28 days of birth from the following general causes: poor maternal health and nutrition, inadequate care during pregnancy and delivery, and lack of essential care upon birth. Specific causes of death include infection, birth asphyxia, birth trauma, and problems relating to premature birth.

Availability and accessibility

In low-income settings, improved availability of appropriate resuscitation equipment and staff trained in its use, is urgently required.

Routine electronic fetal monitoring with ultrasound is widely used to detect fetal problems, but it carries a relatively high false-positive rate and is of questionable clinical benefit. Development of technologies to detect fetal health status that have a low false-positive rate, are easy to use, and operate on boost-chargeable battery power would greatly enhance the effectiveness and efficiency of this tool.

Appropriateness and affordability

The development of affordable, easy to use and robust ventilators for low-income settings could save the lives of critically ill newborns with respiratory insufficiency. Equipment to adjust oxygen flow to meet the precise needs of newborn infants is on the market but not affordable for many settings. Furthermore, a reliable supply of oxygen is often lacking.

Premature infants who need to be referred to a hospital or transferred to another hospital need to be placed in incubators, robust enough to withstand transportation, particularly in the often difficult conditions of low-resource areas. Such transportable incubators exist but are generally too expensive for use in developing countries. Therefore, development of transportable incubators appropriate for use in low-income, rural or semi-rural settings is needed.

Bibliography

Darmstadt GL et al. Evidence-based, cost-effective interventions: how many newborn babies can we save? *Lancet,* 2005, 365(9463):977–988.

Lawn JE, Rudan I, Rubens C. Four million newborn deaths: is the global research agenda evidence-based? *Early Human Development*, 2008, 84 (12):809–814.

Oxygen therapy. In: Woods DL, ed. *Perinatal Education Programme (PEP) - newborn care manual*. International Association for Maternal and Neonatal Health, 2008 (http://www.gfmer.ch/PEP/NCM_Contents.htm, accessed 27 February 2010).

World health report 2005: make every mother and child count. Geneva, World Health Organization, 2005.

6.4.2 Lower respiratory tract infections

Lower respiratory tract infections (LRTIs) encompasses a spectrum of diseases. Caused mainly by viruses or bacteria invading the trachea, bronchi, or lungs, LRTIs are generally more serious than upper respiratory tract infections. Pneumonia remains the leading cause of death in children under five years old worldwide, killing about 2 million children every year, equivalent to one fifth of all child deaths annually. A study on LRTIs in infants under 59 months in 10 developing countries found respiratory syncytial virus (RSV) to be the most common viral cause of LRTIs, with *Streptococcus pneumoniae* (pneumococcus) and *Haemophilus influenzae* the most common bacterial causes. RSV is currently successfully detected by molecular technology, which is expensive and technically challenging.

Availability and accessibility

A pulse oximeter, a device that indirectly measures the oxygen saturation of a patient's blood, is often used to monitor children presenting with symptoms of pneumonia. Coupled with a reliable oxygen supply, this strategy may improve quality of care and reduce child mortality. These technologies are available at low-cost. However, in many developing countries these devices are not being implemented for various reasons, such as maintenance issues and/or lack of information, preventing proper decision-making. Better information is therefore needed to help with procurement and improve recommendations made in clinical guidelines and protocols.

Appropriateness and affordability

Because of clinical guidelines and clinical experience, many clinicians usually treat a suspected LTRI without waiting for diagnostic identification of the specific bacterium responsible. In addition, urgent treatment is often needed to reduce morbidity and mortality. However, in some cases where there may be the possibility of antibiotic resistance and concurrent infection, diagnostic identification may be necessary. Development of affordable diagnostic tests to identify antibiotic resistance may be able to distinguish patients who require alternative treatment.

Bibliography

Duke T et al. Pulse oximetry: technology to reduce child mortality in developing countries. *Annals of Tropical Paediatrics*, 2009, 29(3):165–175.

Klig JE. Current challenges in lower respiratory infections in children. *Current Opinion in Paediatrics*, 2004, 16(1):107–112.

Meer V et al. Diagnostic value of C reactive protein in infections of the lower respiratory tract: systematic review. *British Medical Journal*, 2005, 331(7507):26.

Scott JAG. The global epidemiology of childhood pneumonia 20 years on. *Bulletin of the World Health Organization,* 2008, 86(6):494–496.

Selwyn BJ. The epidemiology of acute respiratory tract infection in young children: comparison of findings from several developing countries. *Reviews of Infectious Diseases,* 1990, 12(Suppl. 8):S870–888.

UK Respiratory Research Foundation – research strategy. International Primary Care Respiratory Group, 2010 (http://www.theipcrg.org/ukrrf/res_strategy.php, accessed 27 February 2010).

6.4.3 Unipolar depressive disorders

According to WHO estimates, depression currently affects about 121 million people worldwide. In 2000, depression was ranked as the leading cause of disability in terms of years lost due to a disability (YLD) and fourth in terms of disability-adjusted life years (DALYs). By 2030, depression is expected to be first in the list of high-burden diseases worldwide in terms of DALYs, for all ages and both sexes.

Availability and accessibility

The management of depression may differ widely between countries and regions, depending on tradition, culture, and means to diagnose and treat the condition. Diagnosis can sometimes be a particular problem. The mainstay of treatment is anti-depressive drug therapy but cognitive behavioural therapy is increasingly being used.

Choosing which specific therapy to use for which patient, at which stage of the condition, in which socioeconomic setting, and for what period of time remains a therapeutic dilemma that requires further research.

Appropriateness and affordability

Evidence of non-drug interventions, such as medical technologies (see below) is difficult to obtain. Therefore, robust evidence of effectiveness on which to base the choice of medical technologies to be used for a specific patient with a particular type of depressive disorder should be collected and published.

Cutting-edge technologies

Cutting-edge technologies are coming to the market in high-resource countries and include deep brain stimulation, web-based cognitive-behavioural therapy, vagus nerve stimulation, transcranial magnetic stimulation, magnetic seizure therapy and transcranial direct-current stimulation. Each approach has its indications, with its reported successes and failures and its advocates and detractors. As yet there is no solid evidence base to support any of these interventions.

Bibliography

Arul-Anandam AP, Loo C. Transcranial direct current stimulation: a new tool for the treatment of depression? *Journal of Affective Disorders,* 2004, 117(3):137–145.

Depression. Geneva, World Health Organization, 2010 (http://www.who.int/mental_health/management/depression/definition/en/, accessed 27 February 2010).

Linden DE. Brain imaging and psychotherapy: methodological considerations and practical implications. *European Archives of Psychiatry & Clinical Neuroscience*, 2008, 258 (Suppl. 5):71–75.

6.4.4 Ischaemic heart disease

Every year, cardiovascular diseases cause about 17 million deaths worldwide, according to WHO estimates. Some 40% are due to ischaemic heart disease (IHD). Approximately 80% of these deaths occur in developing countries. Morbidity and mortality from cardiovascular disease generally, and IHD in particular, are increasing. Behavioural risk factors include an unbalanced diet, reduced physical activity, and smoking. Living longer is also associated with co-morbidity (the presence of several illnesses at the same time) and with chronic debilitating conditions, such as heart disease.

Availability and accessibility

Prevention of IHD is an important goal. Evidence-based preventative measures that can be adapted to local cultures, concepts, and communities could potentially contribute to preventing IHD and its associated disease burden.

Despite the widely accepted view that IHD represents a large public health burden in developing countries, comprehensive epidemiologic data to support this view are generally lacking. Most epidemiological research on this disease has been conducted in high-resource settings. This imbalance hampers attempts by developing country authorities to implement health strategies aimed at curbing the rising burden of IHD, and needs to be addressed. This imbalance also discourages R&D activities on innovative therapeutic technologies applicable worldwide and not, as is currently the case, predominantly in high-resource settings.

Administration of aspirin and anti-thrombotic therapy are of proven benefit, if given as soon as possible after the onset of a myocardial infarction. However, anti- thrombotic therapy is under-utilized in most low-resource settings, because of lacking diagnostic tools like electrocardiographs and cardiac biomarkers. Single channel electrocardiography with interpretation is needed. These electrocardiographs are currently available at an affordable price but are not often used in low-income settings. A possible reason for this under-use is the lack of information on their availability at the decision-making level.

Another major problem is the lack of emergency response units, such as ambulances, that have the appropriate equipment needed to resuscitate and maintain the patient who has had a suspected myocardial infarction. This situation needs to be urgently addressed by the development of affordable, robust, and appropriately-designed emergency equipment.

Appropriateness and affordability

Cardiopulmonary resuscitation devices can be life-saving in cases of cardiac arrest or severe arrhythmias but are inaccessible in most low-resource settings. Therefore, it would be advantageous to the public health needs of low-income settings to develop affordable and robustly designed cardiopulmonary resuscitation equipment, including affordable defibrillators, which are easy to operate (similar to those present in public areas like cinemas and airports in high-income countries).

To avoid long-term effects, diagnosing and monitoring IHD is important. There is a need to develop a kit containing simple and affordable technologies for measuring blood pressure, blood glucose and cholesterol levels to assess cardiovascular risk.

Low-resource countries generally lack medical devices for diagnosing IHD at the primary health-care level and for deciding on referral of a patient to a health-care facility where diagnosis can be established and the patient given appropriate treatment. Accurate, non-invasive technologies to diagnose IHD (such as electrocardiographs that are easy to use, affordable, and can transmit signals to a hospital for assessment by a cardiologist) do exist, but are currently not widely used. Research into the reasons for the lack of uptake of this technology would be useful.

Bibliography

Cardiovascular disease: prevention and control. Geneva, World Health Organization, 2010 (http://www.who.int/dietphysicalactivity/publications/facts/cvd/en/, accessed 27 February 2010).

Commerford P, Ntsekhe M. Ischaemic heart disease in Africa. How common is it? Will it become more common? *Heart,* 2008, 94(7):824–825.

Jafary FH, Ahmed H, Kiani J. Outcomes of primary percutaneous coronary intervention at a joint commission international accredited hospital in a developing country - can good results, possibly similar to the west, be achieved? *Journal of Invasive Cardiology*, 2007, 19(10):417–423.

Lindholm LH, Mendis S. Prevention of cardiovascular disease in developing countries. *Lancet*, 2007, 370(9589):720–722.

Mendis S et al. Recommendations for blood pressure measuring devices for office/clinic use in low-resource settings. *Blood Pressure Monitoring*, 2005, 10(1):3–10.

Nakazawa G et al. A review of current devices and a look at new technology: drug-eluting stents. *Expert Review of Medical Devices*, 2009, 6(1):33–42.

Pais P. Preventing ishaemic heart disease in developing countries. *Evidence-based Cardiovascular Medicine,* 2006, 10(2):85–88.

Prevention of recurrent heart attacks and strokes in low and middle income populations: evidence-based recommendations for policy-makers and health professionals. Geneva, World Health Organization, 2003.

Walker BA, Khandoker AH, Black J. *Low cost ECG monitor for developing countries.* Intelligent sensors, sensor networks and information processing (SSNIP)2009.

6.4.5 Cerebrovascular disease (stroke)

Since many of the risk factors of stroke are similar to those of IHD, cerebrovascular disease is considered next.

Stroke is a sudden interruption in blood supply to the brain and is responsible for about 4.4 million deaths every year. About 75% of strokes result from blockage of the arteries leading to the brain (ischaemic stroke), about 15% from a ruptured blood vessel bleeding into brain tissue (haemorrhagic stroke) and about 10% from bleeding—often from a ruptured aneurysm—(subarachnoid haemorrhage). Common symptoms of stroke include unilateral sudden weakness and loss of sensation, headache, or difficulty speaking, seeing, or walking. The risk of stroke more than doubles each decade after the age of 55. Other risk factors for stroke include hypertension, diabetes, alcohol use, and arterial fibrillation. Fifteen per cent of people who have experienced a cerebrovascular accident die shortly after the event.

Availability and accessibility

Before initiating any treatment, a CT scan is required to establish definitive diagnosis and to ascertain the type of stroke so that the correct treatment can be given. As CT equipment is rarely available to most patients living in low-resource settings, they cannot benefit from definitive diagnosis and appropriate treatment. MRI and CT scans are also of proven value in the diagnosis and localization of injured brain tissue and in identifying brain tissue at risk of injury from stroke. Again, due to the lack of MRI and CT scanners in low-resource settings, people who have experienced a stroke in these areas are at a distinct disadvantage.

Appropriateness and affordability

In many cases, stroke is preventable. However, as with IHD, to assess the risk of stroke, measurements of blood pressure, blood sugar and blood cholesterol must be made which once again emphasizes the need for simple, affordable measuring kits.

Stroke commonly results in functioning problems. Research of devices to assist stroke victims is under way in high-resource countries but has not attained priority in low-resource countries. Therefore, there is a need to develop appropriate assistive products to help restore functional capacity for people disabled by stroke in low-income settings.

Cutting-edge technology

Currently, interventions for stroke are available in high-resource settings, such as thromboembolectomy for acute stroke and stenting of cervical or cerebral arteries to aid stroke prevention. However, conclusive evidence to support the validity of this trend is lacking. Therefore, assessment of the value of these techniques—including clinical evaluation of innovative stents—in preventing cerebral ischaemia or its recurrence—is still required. In addition, assessment of the clinical outcomes of electro-stimulation therapies (supposed to speed up and enhance functional recovery in stroke patients) has not been properly evaluated.

Technologies like rehabilitation robotics are being developed in the rehabilitative treatment of post-stroke patients with upper limb impairment; evaluation of their functional outcomes is under way. Recently developed is the assisted movement with enhanced sensation (AMES) therapy—a new approach for managing brain-injured patients and patients with severe chronic impairments. Although such technologies show promise, their safety and effectiveness have yet to be properly evaluated.

Bibliography

Cordo P et al. Assisted movement with enhanced sensation (AMES): coupling motor and sensory to remediate motor deficits in chronic stroke patients. *Neurorehabilitation & Neural Repair,* 2009, 23(1):67–77.

Masiero S et al. Upper limb rehabilitation robotics after stroke: a perspective from the University of Padua, Italy. *Journal of Rehabilitation Medicine,* 41(12):981–985.

Merrill DR. Review of electrical stimulation in cerebral palsy and recommendations for future directions. *Developmental Medicine & Child Neurology,* 2009, 51(Suppl. 4):154–165.

Package of essential noncommunicable (PEN) disease interventions for primary health care in low-resource settings. Geneva, World Health Organization (in press).

Popovic DB, Sinkaer T, Popovic MB. Electrical stimulation as a means for achieving recovery of function in stroke patients. *Neurorehabilitation,* 2009, 25(1):45–58.

Prevention of cardiovascular disease: guidelines for assessment and management of total cardiovascular risk. Geneva, World Health Organization, 2007.

Prevention of recurrent heart attacks and strokes in low and middle income populations: evidence-based recommendations for policy-makers and health professionals. Geneva, World Health Organization, 2003.

Reid AW, Reid DB, Roditi GH. Imaging in endovascular therapy: our future. *Journal of Endovascular Therapy,* 2009, 16(Suppl 1): 122–41.

Sakai N, Sakai C. Stent for neurovascular diseases. *Review, Brain & Nerve / Shinkei Kenkyu no Shinpo,* 2009, 61(9):1023–1028.

Schneck MJ. Critical appraisal of medical devices in the management of cerebrovascular disease. *Therapeutics and Clinical Risk Management,* 2008, 4(1):19–29.

Singh R et al. Telemedicine in emergency neurological service provision in Singapore: using technology to overcome limitations. *Telemedicine Journal & E-Health,* 2009, 15(6):560–565.

6.4.6 HIV/AIDS

In 2008, an estimated 33 million people were living with HIV infection and 2.0 million died from HIV/AIDS. In some parts of the world, notably southern Africa, between 14% and 28% of the population was infected with the virus in 2007. Over 2 million children under five years old were living with HIV and more than a quarter of a million children died from the infection. HIV/AIDS is projected to decline over the next two decades, and HIV infection has the potential to be managed as a chronic condition, through the use of antiretroviral therapies.

Availability and accessibility

Early detection of HIV infection in newborn infants exposed to the HIV virus is critically important for the clinical management of both mother and infant, particularly in places where breastfeeding is crucial to infant survival. HIV infection in newborns and infants can only be diagnosed with tests that either detect HIV DNA or RNA, as the results of serological tests are confounded by the presence of maternal antibodies to the virus. Therefore, such tests should be based on viral quantification. The development of relatively simple diagnostic tests for early diagnosis of HIV infection in newborn infants and young children would contribute to improved targeted treatment for this group.

Reliable estimates of HIV incidence are critical for epidemiological assessment and to assess the effect of prevention and treatment programmes. Direct measurement of incidence through prospective surveillance studies of HIV-negative people is expensive and difficult to sustain, even for high-resource settings. The development of tests and/or testing algorithms to reliably measure HIV incidence in target populations could provide much needed critical information in a more efficient and affordable manner.

Appropriateness and affordability

There are two types of technologies that are widely used to monitor progression of HIV infection and help in the decision to initiate treatment and monitor its effectiveness. The first measures the level of CD4 + T-cells in the body, which decreases as the HIV infections progresses and provides a measure of the overall immune status. The second technology measures the concentration or viral load of free circulating HIV genomes in the blood of the patient. Although CD4 tests are increasingly available in smaller centres, currently these tests are expensive. In addition, viral load detection is difficult to perform other than in well-equipped reference centres. This hampers the cost-effective use of treatment programmes.

Development of affordable and easy-to-operate CD4 and viral load technologies is therefore required. Such technologies should be easily transportable and adapted to resource-limited settings (e.g. efficacious in hot, humid environments).

Bibliography

2008 report on the global AIDS epidemic. Geneva, Joint United Nations Programme on HIV/AIDS (UNAIDS), 2008 (UNAIDS/08.25E/JC1510E).

Iweala OI. HIV diagnostic tests: an overview. *Contraception,* 2004, 70 (2):141–147.

Cherutich P et al. Optimizing paediatric HIV Care inKenya: challenges in early infant diagnosis. *WHO Bulletin,* 2008,86 (2):155–160.

Ficus SA et al. HIV-1 viral load assays for resource limited settings, *PloS Medicine,* 2006;3(10):1743-1750.

Bush M et al. Beyond detuning: ten years of progress and new challenges in the development and application of assays for HIV incidence estimation from surveys, *AIDS,* 2010 (submitted).

Murphy G, Parry JV. Assays for the detection of recent infections with human immunodeficiency virus type 1. *Euro Surveill* 2008,13:18966.

6.4.7 Road traffic accidents

Every year, road traffic accidents kill an estimated 1.2 million people and injure or disable a further 20–60 million. By 2030, road traffic accidents are expected to become the fourth largest contributor to the burden of disability worldwide. About 90% of road traffic deaths occur in developing countries, where pedestrians, cyclists, and users of two-wheel vehicles (scooters, motorbikes) are the most vulnerable. Bone trauma resulting form fractures due to road traffic accidents can be considered as a major burden of disease. Untreated fractures can lead to severe functional problems, further adding to this burden. Road traffic deaths are likely to increase by more than 80% in developing countries and to decrease by nearly 30% in industrialized countries up to 2030. Road traffic accidents are projected to rise considerably in the African and South-East Asian Regions.

Preventing road traffic accidents is vital: traffic lights, speed control and the use of safety belts are among the measures considered to be most effective.

Availability and accessibility

The lag time between accident and arrival at a health-care facility increases the mortality and morbidity of road traffic accidents. Much of the mortality could be avoided by timely stabilization and medical care, such as endotracheal intubation and resuscitation at the scene of an accident, and timely use of emergency equipment, such as ventilators, tracheal tubes, laryngeal masks, and basic diagnostic tests. Easy-to-use ultrasound devices for diagnosis of internal, especially intra-abdominal bleeding, would also be a useful development.

Training and testing airway devices in pre-hospital emergency settings, in different sizes and in circumstances covering the spectrum of medical care difficulties encountered in road accidents, may counteract any risk associated with intubation.

Emergency care, including imaging techniques to diagnose bone trauma in a health-care facility, is necessary for immediately addressing urgent health issues and to prevent long-term disability. Standard radiology remains the major diagnostic tool. Affordable X-ray equipment has been developed, however, universal access to this diagnostic tool is limited, particularly in low-resource settings. Research into limited uptake may discover the reasons for this deficiency.

Training in surgical and non-surgical early interventions may help to prevent loss of functionality. Based on recent WHO country assessments, surgery is becoming an integral part of primary health care and a cost-effective strategy of dealing with many health challenges specific to resource-poor settings.[1] Development of a self-contained, mobile integrated kit of essential surgical instruments could provide the basic tools necessary for surgical interventions. Such a kit should also be easy to maintain and use on-site.

The delivery of surgical care (including trauma) is highly dependant on the availability of a trained anaesthesia workforce as well as adequate and affordable anaesthesia equipment. While both resources are generally lacking in developing countries, the more serious issue is a lack of equitable services between rich and poor. These deficiencies need to be addressed *(182)*.

Bibliography

Global status report on road safety: time for action. Geneva, World Health Organization, 2009.

---

1   Also see http://www.who.int/eht/sps/en/index.html.

Hazen A, Ehiri JE. Road traffic injuries: hidden epidemic in less developed countries. *Journal of the National Medical Association*, 2006, 98(1):73–82.

Khorasani-Zavareh D et al. Post-crash management of road traffic injury victims in Iran. Stakeholders' views on current barriers and potential facilitators. *BMC Emergency Medicine*, 2009, 9:8.

Mock CN et al. Trauma mortality patterns in three nations at different economic levels: implications for global trauma system development. *Journal of Trauma: Injury, Infection, and Critical Care,* 1998, 44(5):804–814.

Rasouli MR, Nouri M, Rahimi-Movaghar V. Spinal cord injuries from road traffic crashes in southeastern Iran. *Chinese Journal of Traumatology*, 2007, 10(6):323–326.

WHO essential emergency equipment generic list. In: Integrated management for emergency and essential surgical care (IMEESC) tool kit. Geneva, World Health Organization, 2007 (http://www.who.int/surgery/imeesc, accessed 21 July 2010).

6.4.8 Tuberculosis

More than 2 billion people—a third of the world's population and mostly young adults in developing countries—are infected with tuberculosis bacillus (TB). In 2006, there was an estimated 9.2 million new cases of TB and 1.7 million deaths. Asia accounts for more than half of all TB deaths. HIV-infected individuals are highly susceptible to TB and tend to have rapidly progressing disease with a high mortality rate.

Availability and accessibility

The most common method for diagnosing TB in developing countries is direct microscopic detection of acid-fast bacteria in sputum. (Detection by bacterial culture is also available in some large centres.) Direct microscopy generally detects a limited percentage (ranges between 20% up to 75%) of true TB cases, and is particularly problematic in individuals who are co-infected with HIV. Development of rapid, cost-

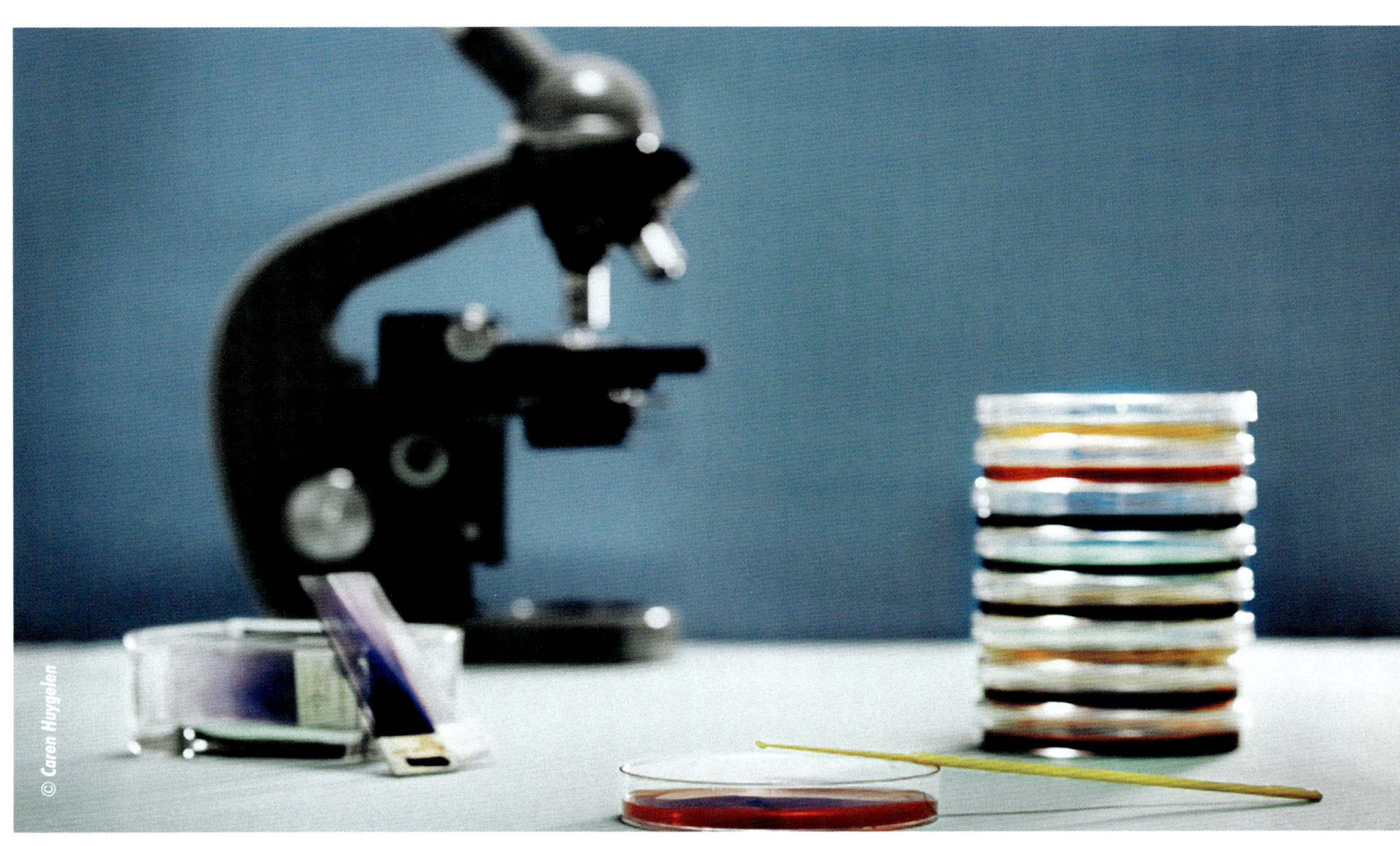

effective and affordable tests for case finding, and guiding therapies that are sufficiently sensitive (to identify infected individuals) and specific (to identify non-infected individuals) are urgently needed.

In order to be able to detect TB at an early stage, a cost-effective test to detect non-symptomatic TB infected people is necessary. Such a test would reduce transmission to other people and allow the early initiation of drug treatment regimens, which in turn could reduce development of drug resistance. Research is needed to determine which tests would meet the conditions of being context-specific and cost-effective in endemic areas.

In many populations, chest X-ray detection of non-symptomatic TB-infected people is currently used for as a first-line screening test. Low-cost chest X-rays have been developed but their accessibility is still limited. Research into the root causes of the limited accessibility of affordable X-ray equipment may help future projects become more successful.

Appropriateness

Traditional bacterial culture, the golden standard for diagnosis of TB, takes four to six weeks to complete and is currently not designed to be used in most areas endemic for the disease. It also requires a physical infrastructure, training and a constant flow of reagents. New, rapid and simple molecular methods to detect TB and TB drug resistance have been developed, but to date these methods have not been widely used. Research into the reasons of their lack of accessibility (which may include inappropriate design and high costs) could contribute to the wider use and uptake of these tests.

Bibliography

Van Cleeff MRA et al. The role and performance of chest X-ray for the diagnosis of tuberculosis: a cost-effectiveness analysis in Nairobi, Kenya. *BMC Infectious Diseases*, 2005, 5:111.

Getahun H et al. Diagnosis of smear-negative pulmonary tuberculosis in people with HIV infection or AIDS in resource-constrained settings: informing urgent policy changes. *Lancet*, 2007, 369(9578):2042–2049.

Global tuberculosis control: epidemiology, strategy, financing. Geneva, World Health Organization, 2009 (WHO/HTM/TB/2009.411).

Improving the diagnosis and treatment of smear-negative pulmonary and extrapulmonary tuberculosis among adults and adolescents: recommendations for HIV-prevalent and resource-constrained settings. Geneva, World Health Organization, 2006.

6.4.9 Malaria

In 2006, 3.3 billion people were at risk of malaria in the 109 countries where the disease is endemic. Nearly half of these countries are in the WHO African Region. Globally, the disease caused an estimated 247 million cases and nearly one million deaths, 85% of them in children under five years old. The African Region accounted for 86% of cases and 91% of deaths, according to WHO estimates.

Availability and accessibility

Diagnosis of bacterial and viral pathogens that cause fever relies primarily on culture methods, which require functioning microbiology laboratories that are often not available in malaria-endemic areas. In many such areas, drug treatment is often given when there is evidence of a history of fever. However, the main causes of febrile illness in malaria-endemic areas cannot be differentiated on the basis of clinical symptoms and signs alone, leading to the over-diagnosis and over-treatment of febrile illness presumed to be malaria, and under-diagnosis and under-treatment of true malaria.

Appropriateness and affordability

Parasitological confirmation by microscopy or rapid diagnostic tests is recommended by WHO in all suspected cases of malaria before treatment is started. However, this recommendation has not been fully implemented. Development of affordable rapid diagnostic tests that allow differentiation between febrile illness due to malaria and that due to other causes would avoid the unnecessary treatment of febrile illness with antimalarial drugs, such as artemesinin combination therapy (ACT), whose overuse could lead to resistance of the main class of drug that is still effective in the treatment of malaria.

In order to ascertain whether a diagnostic test for malaria is appropriate, field validation of antigen-based tests developed for the diagnosis of the main bacterial or viral causes of febrile illness could be performed. Such tests may also help to differentiate between pathogen carriage and invasive infections. In addition, rapid diagnostic tests for malaria are generally not stable at temperatures above 30 degrees Celsius. Development of rapid diagnostic tests that have greater stability at tropical conditions (humidity and high temperatures) would make the test more appropriate for tropical, low-resource settings. Such a test should be manufactured under a stringent quality management system to reduce batch to batch variation.

Bibliography

Elgayoum SME et al. Malaria overdiagnosis and burden of malaria misdiagnosis in the suburbs of central Sudan: special emphasis on artemisinin-based combination therapy era. *Diagnostic Microbiology and Infectious Disease,* 2009, 64(1):20–26.

Endeshaw T et al. Evaluation of light microscopy and rapid diagnostic test for the detection of malaria under operational field conditions: a household survey in Ethiopia. *Malaria Journal*, 2008, 7:118.

Kain KC et al. Imported malaria: prospective analysis of problems in diagnosis and management. *Clinical Infectious Diseases*, 1998, 27(1):142–149.

Murray CK, Bennett JW. Rapid diagnosis of malaria. Review article. *Interdisciplinary Perspectives on Infectious Diseases,* 2009 (http://www.hindawi.com/journals/ipid/2009/415953.html, accessed 27 February 2010).

World malaria report 2008. Geneva, World Health Organization, 2008 (WHO/HTM/GMP/2008.1).

6.4.10 Chronic obstructive pulmonary disease

Chronic obstructive pulmonary disease (COPD) is a life-threatening lung condition. An estimated 210 million people worldwide have COPD and in 2005, 3 million people died of this disease. Nearly 90% of the deaths occurred in developing countries. The primary cause of COPD is tobacco smoke (from tobacco smoking or second-hand smoke).

Spirometry, a technique used to measure lung function, is essential to establish a firm diagnosis of COPD. Currently, spirometers are often unaffordable in low-resource areas. They are also highly sensitive to extreme temperature changes and humidity, and therefore tend not to be reliable in parts of the world affected by these extreme conditions. Moreover, most spirometers require electrical power and are therefore not usable where electricity is not reliably available. Therefore, to enable accurate diagnosis and prognosis of COPD in hot and humid low-resource settings that have intermittent electrical power, it is necessary to develop appropriate portable, affordable spirometry equipment.

Nebulizers convert medications into an air mist that a patient can breathe in through a mouthpiece or mask. However, they are generally not designed for use in the rough conditions found in many low-resource areas, nor are they designed for ease of use and reliability in home-care settings. An alternative to a nebulizer may be a metered dose inhaler (MDI). MDIs are relatively expensive to make, and for this reason they are not often used in resource-poor settings. A cheaper way to produce MDIs would be beneficial. In addition, development of nebulizers designed to function on solar batteries or cells and to be robust enough to withstand difficult conditions in low-resource settings would also be beneficial.

Sometimes, ventilation support is needed for the management of severe exacerbations of COPD. Development of easy-to-use ventilators with built-in compressors and oxygen tank options, designed to be more reliable for use in parts of the world where technical support is lacking, could be a valuable contribution to the management of this disease.

Cutting-edge technology

In high-resource settings design of the nebulizers and oxygen supply should be adapted for home use, with adequate instructions, simple operation, and easy maintenance.

Bibliography

Global strategy for the diagnosis, management, and prevention of chronic obstructive pulmonary disease.

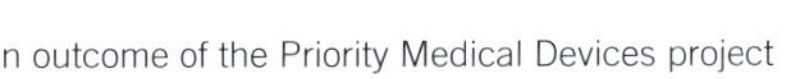

Executive summary, update 2007. Global Initiative for Chronic Obstructive Lung Disease (GOLD), Medical Communications Resources Inc. 2007 (available at http://www.goldcopd.com/Guidelineitem.asp?l1=2&l2=1&intId=996, accessed 12 August 2010).

Wilt TJ et al. *Use of spirometry for case finding, diagnosis, and management of Chronic Obstructive Pulmonary Disease (COPD). Evidence Report/ Technology Assessment No. 121.* Rockville, MD. Agency for Healthcare Research and Quality, September 2005 (AHRQ Publication No. 05-E017-2).

6.4.11 Cataract

Cataract, a clouding of the lens of the eye, is the world's leading cause of blindness. Cataracts are responsible for an estimated 25 million cases of bilateral blindness and 110 million cases of severe visual impairment worldwide. Every year, an additional 1–2 million people become blind as a result of cataracts. As life expectancy increases worldwide, the global public health burden of age-related cataract is likely to grow. Risk factors for age-related cataract include diabetes, prolonged exposure to sunlight, tobacco use and alcohol consumption. Surgical removal of the affected lens and its replacement with an artificial lens (an intraocular lens, IOL) can restore vision in a person with cataract. In 1993, the World Bank rated cataract surgery as one of the most cost-effective health interventions.

Availability and accessibility

Since the increase in the number of people with cataract outpaces the expansion of cataract surgical services in many countries, investing in the training of health-care staff, phacoemulsification equipment, and IOLs may be more beneficial than further research into cutting-edge technologies. Worldwide, approximately 12 million cataract operations are performed annually. However, in order to treat all cataract patients, approximately 16 to 20 million operations a year may be required. Because of the large number of cataract operations, lowering the cost of each intervention could have an impact on cost-effective treatment.

An effective intervention that could have the potential to be widely implemented is the development of a medicinal product that can be injected into the lens, to cause emulsification. This procedure would allow aspiration from the capsule bag, which allows for replacement of the lens by an injectable liquid IOL.

Appropriateness and affordability

Technological ways of offering patients some degree of vision (artificial vision) are in the early investigational stages of research. However, considering the massive current need for treatment in many parts of the developing world, this potential technology is likely to be unaffordable to most people. Therefore, there is an urgent need to develop technologies to provide people with blindness some degree of vision that would be appropriate and affordable for low- and middle- income settings.

New designs and new materials used in the manufacture of IOLs for implantation in patients following cataract surgery are resolving many of the safety problems previously associated with IOL implantation and are expected to increase the use of IOLs. Adapting these designs to make them more appropriate for use in low-resource settings would be a major step forward.

Impaired vision cannot always be resolved by corrective lenses or spectacles, but may be alleviated by adapting the patient's environment. For example, visual aids, such as magnifiers, for people with intractable vision impairment could help to restore functionality.

As with most of the diseases mentioned in this section, prevention is of course the key. There is a cheap and relatively easy way to prevent cataracts that warrants further research—affordable, robust sunglasses that are comfortable to wear and designed in a way that people in different contexts find acceptable to use.

Cutting-edge technology

One limitation of cataract surgery is the unpredictability of the final correction and the risk of residual astigmatism. A possible solution to this problem is the recent development of light-adjustable intraocular lenses, a technology which is currently available mostly in high-resource settings. These lenses contain photosensitive silicone molecules that enable post-operative adjustment of the final refractive power using ultraviolet (UV) light to change the shape of the lenses and therefore their power. Ongoing research to determine whether residual myopia (near-sightedness) and hyper-myopia (in which vision for distant objects is better than for near objects) can be corrected post-operatively by the use of the light-adjustable lens technology is currently under way.

Bibliography

Auffarth GU et al. Design und optische prinzipien von multifokallinsen [Design and optical principles of multifocal lenses]. *Ophthalmologe,* 2008, 105(6):522–526.

Cataract. Geneva, World Health Organization, 2010 (http://www.who.int/topics/cataract/en/, accessed 27 February 2010).

Chayet A et al. Correction of myopia after cataract surgery with a light-adjustable lens. *Ophthalmology*, 2009, 116(8):1432–1435.

Chayet A et al. Correction of residual hyperopia after cataract surgery using the light adjustable intraocular lens technology. *American Journal of Ophthalmology,* 2009, 147(3):392–397.

Facts about cataract. Bethesda MD, National Eye Institute, National Institutes of Health, 2010 (http://www.nei.nih.gov/health/cataract/cataract_facts.asp, accessed 27 February 2010).

Global Initiative for the Elimination of Avoidable Blindness: action plan 2006–2011. Geneva, World Health Organization, 2007.

6.4.12 Hearing loss

According to WHO estimates, in 2005 almost 280 million people worldwide had moderate to profound bilateral hearing impairment. About 80% of these people live in low- or middle-income countries. Infectious diseases such as meningitis, measles, mumps and chronic ear infections can lead to hearing impairment. Head injury or exposure to excessive ambient noise can also cause hearing impairment. Ototoxic drug use at any age, such as certain antibiotics and antimalarial drugs, can also lead to hearing impairments.

Availability and accessibility

Equipment to screen for and diagnose hearing loss early enough to initiate timely intervention, particularly to prevent speech impairment and social exclusion in children, is often too expensive for low-resource countries. Therefore, there is an urgent need to develop practical, robust, affordable and widely-applicable equipment for screening and diagnosing hearing impairment in low-resource settings.

Appropriateness and affordability

Hearing aids and cochlear implants are prohibitively costly in low-resource countries. And as current designs do not allow for long-term use, replacement costs also make these devices out of reach of poorer countries. In addition, batteries for hearing aids are relatively expensive and have a short usable life in hot and humid climates. Follow-up services for hearing aids by trained technicians are also generally costly. Development of longer lasting and more adjustable hearing aids (in addition to longer-lasting batteries for hearing aids used in hot and humid conditions) would be beneficial to people with hearing impairments in low-resource settings.

In addition, hearing aids are generally not designed for use in all age groups. As a result, in low-income settings only 2.5% of people with a hearing impairment who could benefit from a hearing aid actually have one. WHO estimates that global production of hearing aids meets less than 10% of the global need for these devices. Development of appropriately designed and affordable hearing aids and cochlear implants for use in different age groups and contexts is urgently needed.

Bibliography

Cook J et al. Loss of vision and hearing. In: Jamison et al, eds. *Disease control priorities in developing countries*, 2nd edition. Washington DC, IBRD/The World Bank and Oxford University Press, 2006.

Deafness and hearing impairment. Geneva, World Health Organization, 2010 (http://www.who.int/mediacentre/factsheets/fs300/en/index.html, accessed 27 February 2010).

Deafness research UK: Research projects: Cochlear implants. Deafness Research UK, 2007 (http://www.

deafnessresearch.org.uk/?lid=1952, accessed 27 February 2010).

World-wide hearing. WWH, 2007 (http://www. wwhearing.org/, accessed 27 February 2010).

6.4.13 Alcohol use disorders

Globally, alcohol consumption has increased in recent decades, especially in developing countries. Excessive alcohol consumption is known to be a cause of more than 60 types of disease and injury, and according to WHO estimates, accounts for 20–30% of the global incidence of oesophageal cancer, liver cancer, cirrhosis of the liver, homicide, epilepsy, and road traffic accidents. Harmful use of alcohol is also associated with chronic cardiovascular conditions, such as cardiomyopathy, hypertension, coronary artery disease, and stroke. It also increases the risk of acute conditions, such as severe haemorrhage and injuries from traffic accidents or violent behaviour. Worldwide, it is responsible for 1.8 million deaths (3.2% of total deaths) and the loss of 58.3 million years of healthy life.

Availability and accessibility

Gathering accurate national epidemiological data on alcohol consumption requires affordable and accurate methods of measuring individual alcohol consumption. Such tools are currently not widely available, suggesting that further research is required in this area.

It is often difficult to differentiate between patients who have alcohol-induced liver damage from those who have non-alcohol related liver disease, such as viral hepatitis. Ultrasound or other methods of investigating liver size, structure and function may be helpful in identifying people who have alcohol-induced liver damage, but the accuracy of these approaches has yet to be established. The development of accurate technologies in order to differentiate patients who have alcohol induced liver disease from those who have liver disease related to other factors would be a useful aid to diagnosis and ensure correct treatment.

Appropriateness and affordability

Breath analysers for detecting alcohol intoxication represent a growing area of interest due to the serious effects of alcohol intoxication, notably in drivers. Existing tests to detect alcohol levels in blood and urine samples are problematic: their accuracy, particularly in individuals who have consumed other psychoactive substances, is questionable, and their affordability is a barrier to their wider use. Development of accurate, affordable breath analysers that can be used on individuals who have consumed other psychoactive substances in addition to alcohol would help increase wider use of this important test.

Cutting-edge technology

Clinical methods to detect alcohol relapse are available. However, there are no reliable biological tests to detect relapse. Development of alcohol biomarkers to assess and control alcohol consumption and relapse of alcohol dependence would be of great benefit to the management of people who misuse alcohol.

Some individuals may be more susceptible to alcohol than others. Prevention and intervention strategies may be more effective if the role of genetic variation in alcohol-metabolizing enzymes (i.e. genetic susceptibility to alcohol-related disorders) and the role of pharmacogenomics in measuring individual risks could be established.

Bibliography

Bean P et al. Innovative technologies for the diagnosis of alcohol abuse and monitoring abstinence. *Alcoholism: Clinical and Experimental Research,* 2000, 25(2):309–316.

Global status report on alcohol 2004. Geneva, World Health Organization, 2004.

Leung SF et al. Computerized mental health assessment in integrative health clinics: a cross-sectional study using structured interview. *International Journal of Mental Health Nursing,* 2007, 16(6):441–446.

Lucas DL et al. Alcohol and the cardiovascular system research challenges and opportunities. *Journal of the American College of Cardiology,* 2005, 45(12):1916–1924.

Matsumoto I et al. CNS proteomes in alcohol and drug abuse and dependence. *Expert Review of Proteomics,* 2007, 4(4):539–552.

Rehm J et al. Alcohol. In: Jamison et al, eds. *Disease control priorities in developing countries,* 2nd edition. Washington DC, IBRD/The World Bank and Oxford University Press, 2006.

WHO Expert Committee on Problems Related to Alcohol Consumption. Second report. Geneva, Switzerland, 2007 (WHO Technical Report Series, No. 944).

6.4.14 Diabetes mellitus

Diabetes mellitus (particularly type 2) is on the rise across all global regions, with the Americas likely to experience a greater increase over time than other regions. In 2000, when WHO published the latest available estimates, there were 171 million people worldwide with diabetes. About 80% lived in low- and middle-income countries and are primarily in the 45–64-year age group. Every year, about 3 million people die from diabetes, and WHO projects that diabetes deaths are likely to increase by more than 50% in the next 10 years if urgent action is not taken. The projected rise in the prevalence of diabetes is likely to produce a parallel increase in the number of people with diabetic complications such as diabetic retinopathy, diabetic foot disease and peripheral vascular disease. In low- and middle-income countries, less than half of the population with diabetes are actually aware of their condition. This situation can lead to an increased risk of developing serious complications.

Availability and accessibility

Insulin is the main therapy used in managing type 1 diabetes mellitus, but it is also sometimes used in the management of type 2 diabetes. Disposable syringes and needles, to administer the insulin may be too costly for people living in developing countries, especially since the cost of the insulin itself is so high. Auto-disable syringes that eliminate the risk of misuse or infection are not fully used in many areas because of cost, logistical problems of transport, and/or difficult waste disposal. A person requiring insulin for one year would require between 750 and 1000 of these syringes, and supply routes can break down, leaving no safe alternative devices for injecting insulin. Development of methods to simplifying the delivery and safe disposal of auto-disable low-cost syringes may help to reduce the risk associated with reuse of syringes and needles.

Appropriateness and affordability

Diabetes requires regular long-term monitoring. Blood glucose self-monitoring (BGSM) and urine glucose self-monitoring (UGSM) are the main methods used by people living with diabetes to monitor their glucose levels and adjust treatment accordingly. However, very few people in low-resource countries can afford these devices, and the glucose strips required to use these methods are often not accessible. Glucose meters and test strips are generally not adapted to the temperature and humidity extremes common in many low-resource countries. Development of affordable BGSM meters that are better adapted to hot, humid climates and designed for use in low-resource settings is needed. It would also be beneficial if affordable consumables could be included in any future research.

There is evidence that strict control of diabetes may help to prevent many of the complications associated with the disease. However, the means of achieving this control are too costly for many low-resource countries. The most reliable monitoring of glucose in the blood is by measuring glycated haemoglobin HbA1c, a method that is often not readily available in many low-resource settings. Development of reliable, robust and affordable HbA1C monitoring kits would help people with diabetes in low-income settings to better control their condition, which may lead to fewer complications.

In both high- and low-resource countries, blood glucose testing is used by patients at home. Many blood glucose meters require patient with diabetes to insert tiny test strips into the device. The results appear on the display as small numbers. However, as visual problems are common in people with diabetes, the tiny displayed numbers may prevent patients from reading their results. In addition, the design of these devices ignores the fact that at a certain stage of the disease, patients may lose their fine motor skills and therefore have difficulty inserting the test strips. Further development into more appropriate designs could be beneficial to people with diabetes. It would also be helpful if glucose meters that use multiple languages and measurement systems could be developed.

Diabetic foot disease is an increasingly common consequence of diabetes mellitus that may necessitate amputation of the foot if proper care is not provided. Development of orthotic devices to avoid foot amputation in patients with diabetic foot disease, and prosthetic devices for use by patients in whom amputation could not be avoided, would help to increase mobility and avoid functionality difficulties.

Ophthalmoscopes, used to diagnose diabetic retinopathy (and blindness from other causes), are often relatively expensive, so their use in low-resource countries is quite limited. Alternative "smart" high-resolution hand-held ophthalmoscopes that can capture retinal images for digital storage are in the research pipeline but are also likely to be expensive. Therefore, an affordable screening test for diabetic retinopathy that is appropriate for use in low-resource settings would be beneficial.

Cutting-edge technology

Device manufacturers are seeking to further develop automatic insulin delivery systems consisting of an artificial pancreas that uses a glucose sensor to continuously monitor blood sugar levels. In addition, this system could trigger the release of the quantity of insulin needed to keep blood sugar levels within physiological limits, using an implanted pump.

Bibliography

Fox LA et al. A randomized controlled trial of insulin pump therapy in young children with type 1 diabetes. *Diabetes Care,* 2005, 28(6):1277–1281.

Continuous subcutaneous insulin infusion for the treatment of diabetes mellitus (Review of technology appraisal guidance 57). NICE technology appraisal guidance 151. London, National Institute for Health and Clinical Excellence, 2008.

Definition and diagnosis of diabetes mellitus and intermediate hyperglycaemia: report of a WHO/IDF consultation. Geneva, World Health Organization, 2006.

Diabetes action now: an initiative of the World Health Organization and the International Diabetes Federation. World Health Organization/International Diabetes Federation, 2004.

6.5 Future trends in high-burden diseases

6.5.1 Alzheimer disease and other dementias

The term dementia denotes a neurological disorder marked by gradual decline in intellectual functions: memory loss and difficulties in processing information, speaking and making decisions are prominent signs of dementia. Alzheimer disease is the most common form of dementia. Ageing is a key risk factor for dementia but not a direct cause. Population ageing is expected to double the prevalence of dementia over the next 20 years. Currently, an estimated 4.6 million new cases of dementia occur every year worldwide, more than two thirds of which are in low- and middle-income countries. The incapacitating consequences of dementia, its projected escalating prevalence and the absence of proven effective therapies, are likely to place an increasingly heavy burden on caregivers, including family members.

Availability and accessibility

Evidence suggests that early diagnosis of the disease may decrease the chances of developing disabling consequences. However, many symptoms of dementia are difficult to differentiate from those of "normal" ageing. Neurological and other markers of early dementia are promising, but firm evidence is still lacking on the clinical value in people with early, mild cognitive impairment. Diagnostic techniques for dementia are not in widespread use in developing countries.

Several therapies, including a small number of drugs and psychological and behavioural techniques, such as "cognitive training", have shown some benefit in some dementia patients. However, further evidence of their effectiveness is needed before encouraging their widespread use. If proven to be effective, these techniques could be adapted for appropriate use in local low-income contexts.

Cutting-edge technologies

Neurological abnormalities in patients with Alzheimer disease have been demonstrated by imaging technologies, including PET and MRI. However, the precise role of these abnormalities in the pathogenesis of the disease remains unclear and requires further research.

Amyloid imaging has suggested that amyloid levels may be increased in susceptible asymptomatic individuals. However, as yet, there is no evidence of the therapeutic value of this finding, so this area requires further assessment before amyloid imaging can be used as a diagnostic and therapeutic tool.

Video systems can monitor people with early stage dementia. However assessment of the value of home-based video and other telecommunication systems in capturing behavioural patterns symptomatic of dementia without jeopardizing patients' privacy and personal dignity is still required.

There is the potential for "smart" homes—homes that are equipped with high-tech monitoring and feedback technologies—to reduce the dependency of patients with dementia on family and professional caregivers. Smart home systems will need robust monitoring and evaluation to determine the appropriateness, acceptability, and safety of these technologies.

Bibliography

Carrillo MC, Dishman E, Plowman T. Everyday technologies for Alzheimer's disease care: research findings, directions, and challenges. *Alzheimer's and Dementia,* 2009, 5(6):479–488.

Everyday technologies for alzheimer care grant. Chicago, Alzheimer's Association, 2008 (http://www.alz.org/professionals_and_researchers_everyday_technologies_for_alzheimer_care.asp, accessed 18 December 2009).

Ferri CP et al. Global prevalence of dementia: a Delphi consensus study. *Lancet,* 2005, 366(9503):2112–2117.

Mahoneya DF et al. In-home monitoring of persons with dementia: ethical guidelines for technology research and development. *Alzheimer's and Dementia,* 2007, 3(3):217–226.

Schwindt GC, Black SE. Functional imaging studies of episodic memory in Alzheimer's disease: a quantitative meta-analysis. *Neuroimage,* 2009, 45(1):181–190.

6.5.2 Cancer (malignant neoplasms)

According to WHO estimates, in 2008 there were 12.4 million new cancer cases and 7.6 million cancer deaths worldwide. More than half of the cases and 70% of the deaths occurred in developing countries. The most common cancers were lung cancer (1.5 million cases), breast cancer (1.3 million) and colorectal cancer (1.1 million). About 50–60% of cancer patients require radiotherapy, either alone or in combination with chemotherapy and/or surgery.

Availability and accessibility

Diagnosis and treatment of cancer is a sequential, integrated step-by-step process that requires careful planning. In many parts of the world such planning is not possible because of health system weaknesses and infrastructure difficulties. Development of appropriate treatment planning equipment, such as computers and special software with image transfer and viewing capabilities, might overcome problems of patients having to travel from remote areas.

Early diagnosis of cancer improves the outcome of treatment. However, many patients in low-income settings do not have access to early diagnosis. As a result, the majority of patients with malignant neoplasms in developing countries present at a late stage with incurable disease. For example, mammography is an established method to diagnose breast cancer but is not universally accessible. Ultrasound is an essential component of the diagnosis and staging of breast cancer, but is often too costly for low- and middle-income countries. In addition, the training needed to diagnose cancer, such as breast cancer, may be prohibitive. Furthermore, devices needed for investigation, staging and radiotherapy administration—include imaging equipment such as CT scanners, fluoroscopic simulators, PET scanners, single photon emission computed tomography (SPECT) scanners, PET/CT in combination, and nuclear magnetic resonance spectroscopes—are not available or accessible to many patients in low-resource settings.

Therefore, there is a need to develop more reliable, accurate and safe equipment for the early diagnosis and treatment of cancer in low-income settings. Simple, affordable and reliable equipment for early breast cancer detection (e.g. effective automated methods that require less-specialized physicians to review) could also facilitate the expansion of effective diagnosis to more rural areas.

Development of affordable radiotherapy equipment, supported by locally-adapted solutions to make the equipment appropriate for use in low-resource settings and local conditions, would increase the accessibility to appropriate treatment for cancer patients in these areas.

Appropriateness and affordability

For breast cancer, the use of an estrogen receptor assay is critical to the selection of the most appropriate therapy. Its cost, however, is prohibitive in low-resource countries. Development of a reliable and low-cost estrogen receptor assay could potentially increase the effectiveness of the treatment given. The development of robust, affordable ultrasound equipment for the diagnosis and staging of breast cancer, and other soft tissue neoplasms would also be beneficial, but requires the training of health-care professionals to interpret the results.

Cutting-edge technology

Proton therapy—a specific application of radiotherapy—is currently in use in high-resource countries. Creation of a new proton therapy system to treat cancer (at the cost of approximately US$ 25 to US$ 30 million) has recently been launched. However, there is no evidence to support the presence of improved clinical outcomes of proton therapy over conventional radiation modalities. Furthermore, there is an ongoing debate on whether randomized controlled trials are needed to compare the clinical effectiveness of proton therapy versus radiotherapy. The problem is compounded by the fact that traditional radiotherapy systems are available at one thirtieth to one fifth of the price of the newer, more expensive systems, emphasizing the need for clinical outcome studies to be performed for all new technologies.

Bibliography

Barton MB, Frommer M, Shafiq J. Role of radiotherapy in cancer control in low-income and middle-income countries. *Lancet* Oncology, 2006, 7(5):584–595.

Boyle P, Levin B, eds. *World cancer report 2008.* International Agency for Research on Cancer, 2008.
Kanavos P. The rising burden of cancer in the developing world. *Annals of Oncology,* 2006, 17 (Suppl. 8):viii15–viii23.

The World Health Organization's fight against cancer: strategies that prevent, cure and care. Geneva, World Health Organization, 2007.

Valsecchi MG, Steliarova-Foucher E. Cancer registration in developing countries: luxury or necessity? *Lancet Oncology,* 2008, 9:159–167.

Top 10 hospital technology issues: C-Suite watch list for 2009 and beyond. ECRI Institute, 2009.

Goitein M. Should randomized clinical trials be required for proton radiotherapy? *Journal of Clinical Oncology,* 2008, 26(2):175–176.

6.5.3 Osteoarthritis

Osteoarthritis is the most common form of arthritis and a leading cause of disability and pain. Worldwide, nearly 10% of men and 18% of women in their sixties have symptoms of osteoarthritis, 80% have limited movement and 25% have difficulty performing daily activities. Age is the strongest predictor of osteoarthritis and its progression—about 25% of people in their sixties will have X-ray evidence of osteoarthritis. This number increases to nearly 45% for people in their eighties.

In addition to its direct effect on function, osteoarthritis is often associated with other conditions that can adversely affect health, such as obesity and cardiovascular disease. In some cases, osteoarthritis may also be associated with genetic diseases, such as sickle-cell anaemia, or with a nutritional deficiency, such as rickets.

Bone trauma resulting from fractures (e.g. from road traffic accidents, natural disasters, war trauma, and osteoporosis) can lead to post-traumatic osteoarthritis. Therefore, if not properly treated and managed, bone trauma can lead to severe functional disability. Preventative measures to avoid post-traumatic osteoarthritis should be considered a key factor in lowering the global burden of this disease.

Arthoplasty—joint replacement with an artificial implant—remains the main treatment for advanced osteoarthritis.

Availability and accessibility

Standard radiology remains the major diagnostic tool for osteoarthritis. Affordable X-ray equipment has been developed, however, universal access to this diagnostic tool is limited, particularly in low-resource settings. There is some evidence that ultrasonography could be usefully and routinely used to diagnosis and manage osteoarthritis. However, the clinical potential, cost-effectiveness, and ease of use of this technology have not been fully assessed in clinical settings.

Appropriateness and affordability

Artificial implants are usually of limited durability. Further developments in improving the durability of artificial implants may help to preserve function and prevent the costs and complications associated with revision arthroplasty. In addition, improvements in data collection and post-market surveillance are required to improve the biocompatibility of biomaterials used in artificial implants.

There is a need to further develop fracture fixation devices made with affordable material, appropriate to specific contexts, locally developed and produced, to improve functioning and help prevent post-traumatic osteoarthritis.

Functioning problems due to osteoarthritis can often be helped by assistive products. As mentioned frequently throughout this report, there is a serious lack of appropriate assistive products to help overcome functional disabilities. This neglected area requires more research.

Cutting-edge technology

In high-resource settings, there are currently some cutting-edge technologies being developed for the treatment of osteoarthritis, such as cartilage tissue engineering to replace lost cartilage with transplanted stem cells or genetically engineered fibroblast cells. However, robust evidence of the therapeutic effectiveness of these techniques is currently lacking. The concept of biological regeneration using growth factor injection was first proposed in the early 1990s. Since then, the technology to produce recombinant proteins, including growth factors, on an industrial scale has been developed. Currently, the promise of this technology to reduce pain, improve long-term function and prevent early osteoarthritis has yet to be fulfilled.

Bibliography

Handout on health: osteoarthritis. Bethesda MD, National Institute of Arthritis and Musculoskeletal and Skin Diseases, National Institutes of Health, 2006 (http://www.niams.nih.gov/health_info/osteoarthritis/default.asp, accessed 27 February 2010).

Leopold SS. Minimally invasive total knee arthroplasty for osteoarthritis. *New England Journal of Medicine,* 2009, 360 (17):1749–1758.

Masuda K, An HS. Growth factors and the intervertebral disc. *Spine Journal,* 2004, 4(6 Suppl):330S–340S.

Osteoporosis FAQ. Osteoporosis, Australia, 2007 (http://www.osteoporosis.org.au/osteo_faq.php, accessed 27 February 2010).

Tanna S. *Osteoarthritis—opportunities to address pharmaceutical gaps* [Background Paper of Priority Medicines for Europe and the World]. Geneva, World Health Organization, 2004.

6.6 A possible way forward

The purpose of this report has been to identify, inform, and discuss the factors that currently prevent the medical device community (including medical device innovators, choosers, and users) from achieving its full public health potential.

From the examples above, it is clear that there are a lot of possible areas of research to help improve access to appropriate medical devices involved in the high-burden diseases through increasing medical device availability, accessibility, appropriateness, and affordability. The provided examples highlight that although cutting-edge technology to develop new medical devices has its place, research in developing current medical devices to make them appropriate to specific contexts, particularly for low-income settings, is also urgently needed.

The suggested areas of research in this section are only the start of implementing an agenda to improve access to appropriate medical devices. As is best practice, before developing any initiative, the vital process questions of Why? What? How? Who? and When? all need to be answered. This report has gone to great lengths to explain the Why? And the suggested areas of research outlined in this section help provide the basis for the What? But in order to really improve access to appropriate medical devices, the questions of How? Who? and When? need to be answered.

The When? question is relatively easy to answer. Ideally, the implementation of an agenda to improve access to appropriate medical devices should begin as soon as possible. This report has identified and discussed in detail the many problems currently associated with insufficient access to appropriate medical devices, and identified potential solutions to some of these problems. The situation regarding access to appropriate medical devices in high-, middle- and low-income settings is far from ideal. Consequently, there are inadequacies and deficiencies in clinical care and health-care provision that need to be urgently addressed. However, finding practical answers to the questions How? and Who? may be more difficult.

In addition, as discussed in the report and highlighted in the examples that applied the "4 A" questions to medical devices (i.e. Is the medical device Available? Accessible? Appropriate? Affordable?), there are many wide-ranging factors involved in improving access to appropriate medical devices. Research into these factors, such as improved staff training and improved maintenance systems, is also necessary.

This report has also identified the significant deficiencies in access to appropriate assistive products necessary to overcome functioning problems associated with the 15 global high-burden diseases. Any further research in this area— including devising a possible framework to improve the availability, accessibility, appropriateness, and affordability of assistive products—should fully involve communities living with disabilities.

Of course, any further research requires additional funding. With little incentive for companies to invent devices for low-resource markets, the public sector has an important role to play. Partnerships between public sector donors, device manufacturers and the public health sector could share the costs and risks of taking a medical device or an assistive product through the development cycle—design, validation, clinical evaluation, regulatory approval, marketing, distribution and post- market evaluation.

Such public-private-partnerships need to have well-defined needs (such as those outlined in this report), consensus and collaboration to fund, test and promote a product that will respond to local needs. Public-private-partnerships could help to identify and overcome the barriers preventing research on medical devices from being carried out in, and by resource-scarce countries. PATH,[2] an international non-profit organization, is one example of such a partnership. PATH identifies the barriers—low profit margins and regulatory constraints among other things—preventing the technologies that meet public health needs from being widely used in the developing world.

In addition, partnerships between manufacturers in high- and low-resource countries could also foster the creation or strengthening of local research capacity and the establishment of innovation infrastructures facilitated by expertise from manufacturers in industrialized countries.

Although this report has addressed several different areas of concern, the effort to improve global access to medical devices is ongoing and never stagnant. This report is a first step in addressing this important area of work, providing a starting point for future endeavours. Successfully improving access to medical devices in developing countries will require the collaborative effort, dedication, and networking of the many different stakeholders involved. The essential role that medical devices play in health care within high-, middle- and low-income countries, and the significant potential of these technologies to improve the health of populations requires that greater attention and effort be given to this area moving forward.

---

2   http://www.path.org/ (accessed 10 February 2010).

References

1. Lopez AD et al., eds. *Global burden of disease and risk factors.* New York, World Bank and Oxford University Press, 2006.

2. *Landscape analysis: determining the likelihood of any technology corporation developing or adapting technologies for global health purposes using their own funds.* Geneva, World Health Organization, 2010 (in press).

3. *Medical device regulations: global overview and guiding principles.* Geneva, World Health Organization, 2003.

4. Kaplan W, Laing R. *Priority medicines for Europe and the world.* Geneva, World Health Organization, 2004 (WHO/EDM/PAR/2004.7).

5. Free MJ. Achieving appropriate design and widespread use of health care technologies in the developing world. Overcoming obstacles that impede the adaptation and diffusion of priority technologies for primary health care. *International Journal of Gynecology and Obstetrics,* 2004, 85(Suppl. 1):S3–S13.

6. European Commission Directorate-General for Research Directorate. *Responding to global challenges: the role of Europe and of international science and technology cooperation.* Workshop Proceedings Brussels, 4–5 October 2007. European Communities, 2008 (EUR 23614 EN) (http://ec.europa.eu/research/iscp/pdf/workshop_global_challenges_en.pdf, accessed 10 July 2010).

7. Daar AS et al. Top ten biotechnologies for improving health in developing countries. *Nature Genetics,* 2002, 32(2):229–232.

8. *Monitoring financial flows for health research 2009: behind the global numbers.* Geneva, Global Forum for Health Research, 2009.

9. *The 10/90 report on health research 2003/2004.* Geneva, Global Forum for Health Research, 2004.

10. Resolution WHA 60.29. Health technologies. In: *Sixtieth World Health Assembly, Geneva, 14-23 May 2007.*Geneva, World Health Organization, 2007 (WHA60.29 A60/VR/11).

11. *Medium-term strategic plan 2008–2013: progress report.* Programme, budget and administration committee of the Executive Board, Fourth meeting, provisional agenda item 3.2., 11May 2006 (EBPBAC4/4) (http://apps.who.int/gb/pbac/pdf_files/fourth/PBAC4_4-en.pdf, accessed 13 July 2010).

12. Global Harmonization Task Force Study Group 1. *Information document concerning the definition of the term "Medical Device".* The Global Harmonization Task Force, 2005 (GHTF/SG1/N29R16:2005).

13. *Health technologies timeline: greatest engineering achievements of the 20th century.* National Academy of Engineering (http://www.greatachievements.org/?id=3824, accessed 10 July 2010).

14.   Reiser SJ. *Medicine and the reign of technology.* New York, Cambridge University Press, 1978.

15.   Widimsky J. Otto Klein—the forgotten founder of diagnostic cardiac catheterization. *European Heart Journal,* 2008, 29(3):422–423.

16.   Atles LR. *A Practicum for biomedical engineering and technology management issues.* Dubuque, Kendall Hunt Publishing, 2008.

17.   Gaev J. Technology in health care. In: Dyro J, ed. *Clinical engineering handbook.* Burlington, Elsevier Academic Press, 2004:342–345.

18.   Butter M et al. *Robotics for healthcare.* Final Report. European Commission, DG Information Society, 2008.

19.   Grimes SL. The future of clinical engineering: the challenge of change. In: Dyro J, ed. *Clinical engineering handbook.* Burlington, Elsevier Academic Press, 2004: 623–626.

20.   Expert Group on Future Skills Needs. *Future skills needs of the Irish medical devices sector,* 2008 (http://www.skillsireland.ie/publication/egfsnSearch.jsp?ft=/publications/2008/title,2514,en.php, accessed 10 July 2010).

21.   Kohn LT, Corrigan JM, Donaldson MS, eds. *To err is human: building a safer health system.* Washington, National Academies Press, 2000.

22.   Grimes SL. IHE: key to the future of the digital hospital. *Journal of Clinical Engineering,* 2004, 29(4):170–171.

23.   Swedish Institute of Assistive Technologies. *Improved quality of life for persons with diabetes – a proposal to the WHO Advisory Group meeting on innovative technologies,* Singapore, June 20–21, 2009.

24.   Kaplan W et al. *Future public health needs: commonalities and differences between high- and low-resource settings* [Background Paper 8 of the Priority Medical Devices project]. Geneva, World Health Organization (http://whqlibdoc.who.int/hq/2010/WHO_HSS_EHT_DIM_10.8_eng.pdf).

25.   Special report on health care technology. *The Economist,* April 16th 2009.

26.   Geertsma RE et al. *New and emerging medical technologies: a horizon scan of opportunities and risks.* National Institute for Public Health and the Environment (RIVM), 2007 (Report 360020002) (http://www.rivm.nl/bibliotheek/rapporten/360020002.pdf, accessed 13 July 2010).

27.   ECRI Institute. Computer-aided surgery: a GPS for the OR. *Health Devices,* 2009, 38(7):206–218.

28.   *Top 10 hospital technology issues: C-Suite watch list for 2009 and beyond.* ECRI (Emergency Care Research Institute), 2009 (https://www.ecri.org/Forms/Pages/Top_10_Technologies.aspx, accessed 10 July 2010).

29.   California Technology Assessment Forum. *Robot-assisted radical prostatectomy: a technology assessment,* 2008 (http://www.ctaf.org/content/assessment/detail/872, accessed 10 July 2010).

30. *Radiation-emitting products and procedures medical imaging, computed tomography (CT).* Washington DC, United States U.S. Food and Drug Administration, 2002 (http://www.fda.gov/ Radiation-EmittingProducts/RadiationEmittingProductsandProcedures/MedicalImaging/MedicalX-Rays/ ucm115317.htm, accessed 10 July 2010).

31. Carlson D et al. *Trends in medical technology and expected impact on public health.* [Background Paper 7 of the Priority Medical Devices project]. Geneva, World Health Organization.

32. Bougie T et al. *Building bridges between diseases, disabilities and assistive devices: linking the GBD, ICF and ISO 9999* [Background Paper 2 of the Priority Medical Devices project]. Geneva, World Health Organization (http://whqlibdoc.who.int/hq/2010/WHO_HSS_EHT_DIM_10.2_eng.pdf).

33. News release: commitment to strengthen rehabilitation services for people with disabilities. Geneva, World Health Organization, Media centre, May 2005 (http://www.who.int/mediacentre/news/releases/2005/ pr_wha07/en/index.html, accessed 10 July 2010.

34. *Assistive products for persons with disability: classification and terminology.* ISO 9999, fourth edition. National Institute for Public Health and the Environment, (RIVM), WHO Collaborating Centre for the Family of International Classifications (FIC) in the Netherlands, 2007 (http://www.rivm.nl/who-fic/ISO-9999eng.htm, accessed 15 July 2010).

35. MHRA-Medicines and Healthcare products Regulatory Agency. London (http://www.mhra.gov.uk/ Safetyinformation/Generalsafetyinformationandadvice/Technicalinformation/AssistiveTechnology/index. htm, accessed 10 July 2010).

36. Wilcox SB. Applying universal design to medical devices. *Medical Device & Diagnostic Industry,* January 2003 (http://www.mddionline.com/article/applying-universal-design-medical-devices, accessed 10 July 2010).

37. Statement on access to medicines. Geneva, World Health Organization, Media centre, May 2008, (http:// www.who.int/mediacentre/news/statements/2009/access-medicines-20090313/en/index.html, accessed 10 July 2010.

38. Intergovernmental Working Group on Public Health, Innovation and Intellectual Property (IGWG). *The Global Strategy and Plan of Action on Public Health, Innovation and Intellectual Property* (GSPOA). Geneva, World Health Organization, 2008/2009.

39. Wilkinson J. *Medical technology in Europe, 6th March 2009* (http://www.eucomed.org/~/media/7804F 449C2154F8E9207E8E57B19DD4B.ashx, accessed 13 July 2020).

40. Tice JA et al. *Clinical evidence for medical devices: regulatory processes focusing on Europe and the United States of America* [Background Paper 3 of the Priority Medical Devices project]. Geneva, World Health Organization (http://whqlibdoc.who.int/hq/2010/WHO_HSS_EHT_DIM_10.2_eng.pdf).

41. Cheng M. *An overview of medical device policy and regulation.* World Bank, HNP brief. No. 8, February 2007 (http://www-wds.worldbank.org/external/default/WDSContentServer/WDSP/IB/2007/03/02/00031 0607_20070302113845/Rendered/PDF/388190HNPBrief801PUBLIC1.pdf, accessed 13 July 2010).

42. Drummond M, Griffin A, Tarricone R. Economic evaluation for devices and drugs: same or different? *Value in Health*, 2009, 12(4):402–404.

43. Praveenkumar S. *Susceptibility of the European medical device industry amidst economic downturn.* (http://www.frost.com/prod/servlet/market-insight-top.pag?docid=156819802).

44. Gould R, ed. *The world medical markets fact book 2009.* Espicom Business Intelligence, 2009.

45. *3M Healthcare 2008 annual report* (http://solutions.3m.com/wps/portal/3M/en_US/History/3M/Company/financial-facts/annual-report/, accessed 9 February 2010).

46. *Abbott 2008 annual report* (http://www.abbott.com/static/content/microsite/annual_report/2008/index.html, accessed 9 February 2010).

47. *Alcon 2008 annual report* (http://invest.alconinc.com/phoenix.zhtml?c=130946&p=irol-reportsannual, accessed 8 February 2010).

48. B*axter International Inc 2008 report* (http://www.baxter.com/about_baxter/investor_information/annual_report/2008/PDF_files/BaxterAR_2008.pdf, accessed (9 February 2010).

49. *B.Braun 2008 annual report* (http://www.bbraun.com/cps/rde/xchg/bbraun-com/hs.xsl/download-center.html, accessed 9 February 2010).

50. *Beckman Coulter 2008 annual report* (http://phx.corporate-ir.net/phoenix.zhtml?c=64256&p=irol-reportsannual, accessed 9 February 2010).

51. *Becton, Dickinson and Company 2008 annual report* (http://www.annualreports.com/Company/2822, accessed 9 February 2010).

52. *Biomet 2008 annual report* (http://www.biomet.com/corporate/investors/financials/annual.cfm, accessed 9 February 2010).

53. *Boston scientific 2008 annual report* (http://library.corporate-ir.net/library/62/622/62272/items/329935/A4BAD1E1-45B9-4058-AE8B-B37F981220AE_BSX2008AnnualReport.pdf, accessed 9 February 2010).

54. *Cardinal Health 2008 annual report* (http://library.corporate-ir.net/library/10/105/105735/items/311652/102108_CAH_Annual_Report_Form_10-K.pdf, accessed 9 February 2010).

55. *Covidien 2008 annual report* (http://investor.covidien.com/phoenix.zhtml?c=207592&p=irol-reportsannual, accessed 8 February 2010).

56. *C.R. Bard 2008 annual report* (http://www.annualreports.com/HostedData/AnnualReports/PDFArchive/bcr2008.pdf, accessed 9 February 2010).

57. *Danaher 2008 annual report* (http://www.danaher.com/investors/proxy_annual_report.html, accessed 9 February 2010).

58. *Dentsply 2008 annual report* (http://www.dentsply.com/assets/investors/DentsplyAnnualReport.pdf, accessed 9 February 2010).

59. *Dräger 2008 annual report* (http://www.draeger.com/GC/en/investor_relations/financial_reports/, accessed 9 February 2010).

60. *Fresenius Medical Care 2008 annual report* (http://reports.fmc-ag.com/reports/fmc/annual/2008/gb/ English/0/home.html, accessed 9 February 2010).

61. *We are GE 2008 annual report* (http://www.ge.com/investors/financial_reporting/annual_reports.html, accessed 9 February 2010).

62. *Hospira 2008 annual report* (http://www.hospirainvestor.com/phoenix.zhtml?c=175550&p=irol-reportsAnnual, accessed 9 February 2010).

63. *Johnson and Johnson 2008 annual report* (http://www.investor.jnj.com/annual-reports.cfm, accessed 9 February 2010).

64. *Medtronic 2008 annual report* (http://www.medtronic.com/investors/annual-reports/, accessed 8 February 2010).

65. *Olympus 2008 annual report* (http://www.olympus-global.com/en/corc/ir/annualreport/2008/, accessed 9 February 2010).

66. *Philips healthcare 20008 annual report* (http://www.annualreport2008.philips.com/downloads/index. asp, accessed 8 February 2010).

67. *Siemens annual report 2008* (https://w1.siemens.com/annual/08/pool/downloads/pdf/en/pdf_e08_00_ gb2008.pdf, accessed 9 February 2010).

68. *Smith & Nephew annual report 2008* (http://annualreport2008.smith-nephew.com/, accessed 9 February 2010).

69. *Synthes 2008 financial report* (http://www.synthes.com/html/News-Details.8013.0.html?&tx_ synthesnewsbyxml_pi1%5BshowUid%5D=19, accessed 9 February 2010).

70. *St Jude Medical 2008 annual report* (http://www.sjm.com/companyinformation/investorrelations. aspx?section=AnnualReports, accessed 9 February 2010).

71. *Stryker 2008 annual report* (http://www.annualreports.com/Company/2822, accessed 9 February 2010).

72. *Terumo annual report 2008* (http://www.terumo.co.jp/archive/ar_e/AnnualReport_2008_E.pdf, accessed 9 February 2010).

73. *Varian 2008 annual report* (http://varian.investorroom.com/index.php?s=120, accessed 9 February 2010).

74. *Zimmer 2008 annual report* (http://investor.zimmer.com/annuals.cfm?id=8, accessed 9 February 2010).

75. Young JH. The long struggle for the law. Washington DC, United States U.S. Food and Drug Administration, 2009 (http://www.fda.gov/AboutFDA/WhatWeDo/History/CentennialofFDA/TheLongStrugglefortheLaw/ default.htm, accessed 10 July 2010).

76. Ballentine C. Taste of raspberries, taste of death: the 1937 elixir sulfanilamide incident. *FDA Consumer Magazine,* 1981, June Issue.

77.   Melpolder A, Widman A, Doroshow J. *The bitterest pill: how drug companies fail to protect women and how lawsuits save their lives.* New York, Center for Justice and Democracy, 2008.

78.   *The role of medical devices and equipment in contemporary health care systems and services.* World Health Organization. Technical discussion document for the Fifty-third Regional Committee for the Eastern Mediterranean, Agenda item 7 (b), June 2006 (EM/RC53/Tech.Disc.2).

79.   Hamburg MA, Sharfstein JM. The FDA as a public health agency. *New England Journal of Medicine,* 2009, 360:2493–2495.

80.   *Recast of the medical devices directives: public consultation.* Brussels, European Commission, 2008.

81.   *Medical device regulations: global overview and guiding principles.* Geneva, World Health organization, 2003 (http://www.who.int/medical_devices/publications/en/MD_Regulations.pdf, accessed 13 July 2010).

82.   Medical device regulations in Europe (Countries A to M). *Journal of Medical Device Regulation,* November 2007.

83.   Medical device regulations in Europe (Countries N to Z). J*ournal of Medical Device Regulation*, April 2008.

84.   Medical device regulations in Asia, Africa and the Middle East. *Journal of Medical Device Regulation,* April 2007.

85.   Medical Device Regulatory Requirements in China and Hong Kong. *Journal of Medical Device Regulation,* June 2008.

86.   Brolin S. *Global regulatory requirements for medical devices* [thesis]. Eskilstuna, Mälardalen University, 2008.

87.   Petkova H et al. *Barriers to innovation in the field of medical devices* [Background Paper 6 of the Priority Medical Devices project]. Geneva, World Health Organization (http://whqlibdoc.who.int/hq/2010/WHO_HSS_EHT_DIM_10.6_eng.pdf).

88.   Roberts E. Influences on innovation: extrapolations to biomedical technology. In: Roberts E et al, eds. *Biomedical innovation.* Massachusetts, Massachusetts Institute of Technology Press, 1981.

89.   Eastern Research Group. *Unique identification for medical devices—final report.* U.S. Food and Drug Administration, 2006.

90.   Rogers EM. *Diffusion of innovations,* 4th ed. New York, Free Press, 1995.

91.   Szpisjak DF et al. Oxygen consumption of a pneumatically controlled ventilator in a field anesthesia machine. *Anesthesia and Analgesia*, 2008, 107(6):1907–1911.

92.   Hansen J et al. *A stepwise approach to identify gaps in medical devices (Availability Matrix and survey methodology)* [Background Paper 1 of the Priority Medical Devices project]. Geneva, World Health Organization (http://whqlibdoc.who.int/hq/2010/WHO_HSS_EHT_DIM_10.1_eng.pdf).

93.   Sharan P et al. Mental health research priorities in low- and middle-income countries of Africa, Asia, Latin America and the Caribbean. *British Journal of Psychiatry,* 2009, 195(4):354–363.

94.   *The global burden of disease: 2004 update.* Geneva, World Health Organization, 2008.

95.   *Global health risks: mortality and burden of disease attributable to selected major risks.* Geneva, World Health Organization, 2009.

96.   *Disability and rehabilitation. WHO Action plan 2006–2011.* Geneva, World Health Organization, (http://www.who.int/disabilities/publications/dar_action_plan_2006to2011.pdf, accessed 13 July 2010).

97.   I*nternational classification of functioning, disability and health (ICF)*, Geneva, World Health Organization, 2007 (http://www.who.int/classifications/icf/en/, accessed 10 July 2010).

98.   *Rights and dignity of persons with disability.* UN convention on rights of persons with disabilities. United Nations, 2006 (http://www.un.org/disabilities/default.asp?navid=13&pid=150, accessed 10 July 2010).

99.   *International statistical classification of diseases and related health problems* (ICD10). Geneva, World Health Organization, 2007 (http://www.who.int/classifications/icd/en/, accessed 22 March 2010).

100   *World health statistics 2009.* Geneva, World Health Organization, 2009.

101.   Department of Economic and Social Affairs, Population Division. *World population ageing, 1950–2050.* New York, United Nations, 2002 (ST/ESA/SER.A/207).

102.   Rosenberg L, Bloom D. Global demographic trends. *Finance & Development,* 2006, 43(3) (http://www.imf.org/external/pubs/ft/fandd/2006/09/picture.htm, accessed 13 July 2010).

103.   *State of the world population 2007: unleashing the potential of urban growth.* New York, United Nations Population Fund, 2007.

104.   *The world health report 2006: working together for health.* Geneva, World Health Organization, 2006.

105.   *Global status report on road safety.* Geneva, World Health Organization, 2009 (http://whqlibdoc.who.int/hq/2010/WHO_HSS_EHT_DIM_10.7_eng.pdf).

106.   Department of Economic and Social Affairs, Population Division. *World urbanization prospects: the 2007 revision highlights.* New York, United Nations, 2008 (ESA/P/WP/205).

107.   *The world health report 2008: primary health care, now more than ever.* Geneva, World Health Organization, 2008.

108.   *Everybody business: strengthening health systems to improve health outcomes: WHO's framework for action.* Geneva, World Health Organization, 2007.

109.   *The global shortage of health workers and its impact, Fact sheet 302.* Geneva, World Health Organization, 2006 (http://www.who.int/mediacentre/factsheets/fs302/en/, accessed 10 July 2010).

110. Matthews E, Gheerawo R, West J. Academia and industry: managing knowledge transfer to improve patient safety. In: *Proceedings of the International DMI Education Conference, Design Thinking: new challenges for designers, managers and organisations,* Cergy-Pointoise, France, 14–15 April 2008 (http://www.hhc.rca.ac.uk/cms/files/AcademiaAndIndustryJWEMRG.pdf, accessed 10 July 2010).

111. McKelvey M. *Health biotechnology: emerging business models and institutional drivers.* OECD International futures project on "The bioeconomy to 2030: designing a policy agenda". OECD International Futures Programme, 2008.

112. Petkova H. *How gene tests travel: bi-national comparison of the institutional pathways taken by diagnostic genetic testing for maturity onset diabetes of the young (MODY) through the British and the German health care system* [thesis]. Exeter, University of Exeter, 2008.

113. Barcelona European Council. *Presidency conclusions 15 and 16 March 2002* (SN 100/1/02 REV 1) (http://ec.europa.eu/invest-in-research/pdf/download_en/barcelona_european_council.pdf, accessed 13 July 2010).

114. Pammolli F et al. *Medical devices competitiveness and impact on public health expenditure.* Brussels, Entreprise Directorate-General, European Commission, 2005.

115. *Exploratory process on the future of the medical devices sector.* Brussels, European Commission, Consumer Affairs (http://ec.europa.eu/enterprise/sectors/medical-devices/competitiveness/exploratory-process/index_en.htm (accessed 24 June 2010).

116. Hogan S. Seventh Framework Programme Health Theme and SME participation presentation. In: *Proceedings of SMEs in health research—maximising outcomes of EU funded research projects—tools for success. Part I—introduction and objectives FP7 and health.* Brussels, 26 February 2009 (http://cordis.europa.eu/fp7/health/sme_en.html, accessed 10 July 2010).

117. Klaver DL. Heel veel PET- scanners (Many PET-scanners). *Mediator,* 2007, 18(2) (http://www.zonmw.nl/nl/organisatie/publicaties/mediator/archief/mediator-2007/mediator-2-2007/heel-veel-pet-scanners/, accessed 10 July 2010).

118. Feldman MD et al. Who is responsible for evaluating the safety and effectiveness of medical devices? The role of independent technology assessment. *Journal of General Internal Medicine,* 2008, 23(Suppl. 1):57–63.

119. Schreyögg J, Baumlerb B, Busseb R. Balancing adoption and affordability of medical devices in Europe. *Health Policy,* 2009, 92(2):218–224.

120. Brown SL, Bright RA, Travis DA, eds. *Medical device epidemiology and surveillance.* Chichester, Wiley, 2007.

121. Riaño J, Hodess R. *Bribe payers index 2008.* Berlin, Transparency International, 2008.

122. Transparency International. *Global corruption report 2006.* London, Pluto Press, 2006.

123. Nordberg C, Vian T. *Corruption in the health sector (Updated November 2008).* U4 Anti-Corruption Resource Centre, 2008 (U4 ISSUE 7:2008).

124. Perlman L. Shed light on 'physician preference': full disclosure needed in light of secret deals between docs, device makers. *Modern Health Care,* 2007, 37(50):23.

125. Purchasing physician preference items: the search for a cure. *Knowledge@W.P. Carey*, July 18, 2007 (http://knowledge.wpcarey.asu.edu/article.cfm?articleid=1446#, accessed 10 July 2010).

126. McGinnity E. Managing the cost of physician preference items: if you keep doing what you're doing, you'll keep getting what you're getting. *Healthcare Purchasing News*, Nov 2003 (http://findarticles.com/p/articles/mi_m0BPC/is_11_27/ai_110526962/, accessed 10 July 2010).

127. *Innovation, value and collaboration: the European medical technology industry activity report 2007– 2008.* Brussels, Eucomed, 2008 (http://www.eucomed.com/press/~/media/31A9CAFDBD184A0 BB580046396166956.ashx, accessed 13 July 2010).

128. *Assessing the efficacy and safety of medical technologies.* Washington DC, Office of Technology Assessment, 1978 (http://www.fas.org/ota/reports/7805.pdf, accessed 13 July 2010).

129. *The growth in diagnostic imaging utilization.* Pennsylvania Health Care Cost Containment Council, 2004 (http://www.phc4.org/reports/FYI/fyi27.htm, accessed 10 July 2010).

130. Malkin RA. Barriers for medical devices for the developing world. *Expert Review of Medical Devices,* 2007, 4(6):759–763.

131. Malkin RA. Design of health care technologies for the developing world. *Annual Review of Biomedical Engineering*, 2007, 9:567–587.

132. Houngbo PT et al. Policy and management of medical devices for the public health care sector in Benin. *IET Digest*, 2008, 12213:2.

133. Harris G. Crackdown on doctors who take kickbacks. *New York Times,* March 4, 2009 (http://www.nytimes.com/2009/03/04/health/policy/04doctors.html, accessed 10 July 2010).

134. Counterfeit medical products. In: S*ixty-first World Health Assembly A61/16 11.13,* Geneva, 7 April 2008. Geneva, World Health Organization, 2008 (A61/16).

135. Global Programme on Evidence for Health Policy. *Guidelines for WHO guidelines.* Geneva, World Health Organization, 2003 (EIP/GPE/EQC/2003.1).

136. McAlister FA et al. How evidence-based are the recommendations in evidence-based guidelines? *Plos Medicine*, 2007, 4(8):e250.

137. Cabana MD et al. Why don't physicians follow clinical practice guidelines? A framework for improvement. *The Journal of the American Medical Association* 1999, 282(15):1458–1465.

138. Hirsh J, Guyatt G. Clinical experts or methodologists to write clinical guidelines? *Lancet*, 2009, 374(9686):273–275.

139. Global Harmonization Task Force Study Group 1. E*ssential principles of safety and performance of medical devices.* The Global Harmonization Task Force, 2005 (GHTF/SG1/N41R9:2005).

140. Global Harmonization Task Force Study Group 1. *Principles of medical devices classification*. The Global Harmonization Task Force, 2006 (GHTF/SG1/N15:2006).

141. Global Harmonization Task Force Study Group 1. *Principles of conformity assessment for medical devices*. The Global Harmonization Task Force, 2006 (GHTF/SG1/N40:2006).

142. Global Harmonization Task Force Study Group 5. *Clinical evidence: key definitions and concepts*. The Global Harmonization Task Force, 2007 (GHTF/SG5/N2R8:2007).

143. Global Harmonization Task Force Study Group 5. *Clinical evaluation*. The Global Harmonization Task Force, 2007 (GHTF/SG5/N2R8:2007).

144. Hanney S. An assessment of the impact of the NHS Health technology assessment programme. Executive summary, *Health Technology Assessment*, 2007, 11(53).

145. Goodman CS. HTA 101: *introduction to health technology assessment*. The Lewin Group, 2004 (http://www.nlm.nih.gov/nichsr/hta101/hta101.pdf, accessed 13 July 2010).

146. *Multi country regional pooled procurement of medicines. Meeting report, 15–16 January 2007*. Geneva World Health Organization, 2007 (WHO/TCM/MPM/2007.1) (http://www.who.int/medicines/publications/PooledProcurement.pdf, accessed 13 July 2010).

147. *Integrated healthcare networks market overview*. Trumbull CT, Knowledge Source Healthcare market information, 2009, http://knowsource.ecnext.com/coms2/summary_0233-236_ITM, accessed 13 July 2010).

148. *Eucomed contribution to the public consultation of the European Commission in the context of the study on distribution channels for medical devices: combating counterfeit medical devices and safe medical devices in the distribution chain*. Brussels, Eucomed, 2008. (http://www.eucomed.be/press/~/media/441825195F8B46CE859EBE57FCD7A58D.ashx, accessed 13 July 2010).

149. *Recast of the medical devices directives: public consultation*. Brussels, European Commission, 2008.

150. Beenkens F et al. *Context dependency of medical devices* [Background Paper 5 of the Priority Medical Devices project]. Geneva, World Health Organization (http://whqlibdoc.who.int/hq/2010/WHO_HSS_EHT_DIM_10.5_eng.pdf).

151. Dyro J. Donation of medical device technologies. In: Dyro J, ed. *Clinical engineering handbook*. Burlington, Elsevier Academic Press, 2004:155–158.

152. *Guidelines for health care equipment donations*. Geneva, World Health Organization, 2000 (WHO/ARA/97.3).

153. Green M. *Medical equipment: good design or bad design?* Visual Expert Human Factors (http://www.visualexpert.com/Resources/mederror.html, accessed 10 July 2010).

154. Burlington B. *Human factors and the FDA's goals: improved medical device design*. Washington DC, United States, U.S. Food and Drug Administration, 2009 (http://www.fda.gov/MedicalDevices/DeviceRegulationandGuidance/PostmarketRequirements/HumanFactors/ucm126025.htm, accessed 10 July 2010).

155. Dankelman J et al. *Increasing complexity of medical technology and consequences for training and outcome of care* [Background Paper 4 of the Priority Medical Devices project]. Geneva, World Health Organization (http://whqlibdoc.who.int/hq/2010/WHO_HSS_EHT_DIM_10.4_eng.pdf).

156. *Reducing error through design.* Human Factors MD (http://www.humanfactorsmd.com/hfandmedicine_reducerror_design.html, accessed 10 July 2010).

157. Geddes LA. Medical devices: failure modes, accidents, and liability. In: Dyro J, ed. *Clinical engineering handbook.* Burlington, Elsevier Academic Press, 2004:355–358.

158. *Risico's van medische technologie onderschat [Risks from medical technology underestimated].* The Hague, Dutch Health Inspectorate, 2008.

159. *Informal consultation on clinical use of oxygen. Meeting report, 2–3 October 2003.* Geneva, World Health Organization, 2004 (http://www.who.int/surgery/collaborations/Oxygen_Meeting_Report_Geneva_2003.pdf, accessed 13 July 2010).

160. Scottish Health Care Supplies. *Equipment for lifting people: configuration, use and maintenance issues.* Edinburgh, NHS Scotland, 2007 (SAN (SC) 07/32) (http://www.hfs.scot.nhs.uk/online-services/incident-reporting-and-investigation-centre-iric/safety-action-notices-sans/sans-issued-in-2007/, accessed 10 July 2010).

161. *About human factors.* Washington DC, United States, U.S. Food and Drug Administration, 2009 (http://www.fda.gov/MedicalDevices/DeviceRegulationandGuidance/PostmarketRequirements/HumanFactors/ucm119185.htm, accessed 10 July 2010).

162. *Increasing access to health workers in remote and rural areas through improved retention. Global policy recommendations.* Geneva, World Health Organization, 2010.

163. Consoli D et al. The process of health care innovation: problem sequences, systems and symbiosis. In: *Proceedings of technology, innovation and change in health and healthcare.* Geneva, 18–19 October, 2007 (accessed via conference attendance by researcher personally).

164. Hopkins M. *Technique-led technological change and the 'hidden research system': genetic testing in the NHS* [thesis]. Brighton, University of Sussex, 2004.

165. Greenhalgh T et al. *Diffusion of innovations in health service organizations: a systematic literature review.* London, BMJ books, 2005.

166. Ford GS, Koutsky TM, Spiwak LJ. *A valley of death in the innovation sequence: an economic investigation.* Prepared for the Commerce Department, Technology Administration, 2007 (http://ssrn.com/abstract=1093006, accessed 10 July 2010).

167. Tsu V, Shane B. New and underutilized technologies to reduce maternal mortality: call to action from a Bellagio workshop. *International Journal of Gynecology and Obstetrics*, 2004, 85(Suppl. 1): S83–S93.

168. International Organization for Standardization. *ISO action plan for developing countries 2005–2010.* Geneva, ISO Central Secretariat, 2005 (http://www.iso.org/iso/actionplan_2005.pdf, accessed 10 July 2010).

169.   Hofstede G. *Culture's consequences: international differences in work-related values.* Beverley Hills, Sage, 1984.

170.   Barlow J, Bayer S, Curry R. Implementing complex innovations in fluid multi-stakeholder environments: experiences of 'telecare'. *Technovation*, 2006: 26(3):396–406.

171.   Lister M. Transfer of medical technology to developing countries. *Indian Journal for the Practising Doctor,* 2004, 1(2):69–74.

172.   Hotchkiss R. *Wheelchair for the third world in new medical devices: Invention, development and use.* Washington DC, National Academy of Engineering, 1988.

173.   Meier B. Costs surge for medical devices, but benefits are opaque. *New York Times*, 4 November 2009 (http://www.nytimes.com/2009/11/05/business/05device.html?_r=1&scp=2&sq=defibrillators&st=cse, accessed 10 July 2010).

174.   Prahalad CK. *The fortune at the bottom of the pyramid: eradicating poverty through profits.* Upper Saddle River, Wharton School Publishing, 2006.

175.   Arya AP, Klenerman L. The Jaipur foot. *Journal of Bone and Joint Surgery, 2008,* British Volume 90-B (11):1414–1421.

176.   Drury P. The eHealth agenda for developing countries. *World Hospitals and Health Services*, 2005, 41(4):38–40.

177.   Salicrup LA, Fedorkova L. Challenges and opportunities for enhancing biotechnology and technology transfer in developing countries. *Biotechnology Advances*, 2006, 24(1):69–79.

178.   Gelijns A, Rosenberg N. The dynamics of technological change in medicine. *Health Affairs*, 1994, 13(3):28–46.

179.   Lungen M et al. Using diagnosis-related groups: the situation in the United Kingdom NHS and in Germany. *European Journal of Health Economics,* 2004, 5 (4):287–289.

180.   Maurice J. Restoring sight to the millions: the Aravind way. *Bulletin of the World Health Organization* [online], 2001, 79 (3):270–271 (http://www.scielosp.org/scielo.php?script=sci_arttext&pid=S0042-96862001000300022&lng=en&nrm=iso, accessed 10 July 2010).

182.   Cherian M et al. Building and retaining the neglected anaesthesia health workforce: is it crucial for health systems strengthening through primary health care? *Bulletin of the World Health Organization,* online first (http://www.who.int/surgery/Buildingtheanaesthesiahealthworkforce.pdf, accessed 13 July 2010).

183.   WHO essential emergency equipment generic list. In: *Integrated management for emergency and essential surgical care (IMEESC) tool kit.* Geneva, World Health Organization, 2007 (http://www.who.int/surgery/imeesc, accessed 21 July 2010).

Glossary

Accessibility: refers to people's ability to obtain and appropriately use good-quality health technologies when they are needed.

Adverse event: any untoward medical occurrence in a subject whether it is device-related or not.

Affordability: in the context of this report it is defined as the extent to which the intended clients of a service can pay for it.

Appropriate(ness): refers to medical methods, procedures, techniques, and equipment that are scientifically valid, adapted to local needs, acceptable to both patient and health-care personnel, and that can be utilized and maintained with resources the community or country can afford.

Availability: when a medical device can be found on the medical device market.

Benchmarking: a process of measuring another organization's product or service according to specified standards in order to compare it with and improve one's own product or service.

Best practice: an examination of the methods by which optimal outcomes are achieved.

Care pathways: one mechanism of putting a protocol into operation. Care pathways determine locally agreed, multidisciplinary practice, based on guidelines and evidence (where available) for a specific patient group. They form all, or part of the clinical record, they document the care given, and they facilitate the evaluation of outcomes for quality improvement purposes.

Clinical evaluation: the assessment and analysis of clinical data pertaining to a medical device in order to verify the clinical safety and performance of the device.

Clinical evidence: the clinical data and the clinical evaluation report pertaining to a medical device.

Clinical guideline: systematically-developed statements to assist practitioner and patient decisions about appropriate health care for specific clinical circumstances. A clinical guideline is a tool to support clinical decision-making and it covers a specific clinical problem.

Conformity assessment: systematic examination of evidence generated and procedures undertaken by the manufacturer, under requirements established by a regulatory authority, to determine that a medical device is safe and performs as intended by the manufacturer and, therefore, conforms to the Essential Principles of Safety and Performance for medical devices.

Conformity assessment body (CAB): a body engaged in the performance of procedures for determining whether the relevant requirements in technical regulations or standards are fulfilled. A CAB is authorized to undertake specified conformity assessment activities by a regulatory authority that will ensure performance of the CAB is monitored and, if necessary, withdraw designation.

Consumables: liquids or supplies required for the use of the equipment but allowing only limited, or no, reuse.

Core set: an ICF core set is a selection of ICF classes representing relevant aspects in the functioning of people with a specific disease or health problem.

Cost(s): (1) the value of the resources used in an activity; (2) the benefits sacrificed through a particular event or choice of action rather than another.

Cost-effectiveness analysis: analysis which involves the allocation of scarce resources among competing alternative uses, and the distribution of the products from these uses among the members of the society.

DALY (disability-adjusted life year): one DALY can be thought of as one lost year of "healthy" life. The sum of these DALYs across the population, or the burden of disease, can be thought of as a measurement of the gap between current health status and an ideal health situation where the entire population lives to an advanced age, free of disease and disability.

Effectiveness: a device is clinically effective when it produces the effect intended by the manufacturer relative to the medical condition for which it was created.

Efficacy: the ability to produce a desired or intended result, as linked to the performance of a device.

eHealth: the use of information and communication technologies (ICT) for health.

Equity in health: where people's needs guide the distribution of resources and opportunities for well-being.

Gap: a disparity between health-care need and reality.

Global burden of disease (GBD): the WHO GBD project draws on a wide range of data sources to quantify global and regional effects of diseases, injuries and risk factors on population health.

Hazard: potential cause of harm.

Health care: any type of service provided by professionals or paraprofessionals with an impact on health status.

Health technology: the application of organized knowledge and skills in the form of devices, medicines, vaccines, procedures, and systems developed to solve a health problem and improve quality of lives.

Health technology assessment (HTA): the systematic evaluation of properties, effects and/or impacts of health-care technology. HTA defines a multidisciplinary activity that systematically examines technical performance, safety, clinical efficacy and effectiveness, cost, cost-effectiveness, organizational impact, social consequences, and legal and ethical aspects of the application of a health technology.

Medical device: any instrument, apparatus, implement, machine, appliance, implant, in vitro reagent or calibrator, software, material or other similar or related article:
a) intended by the manufacturer to be used, alone or in combination, for humans for one or more of the specific purpose(s) of:
- diagnosis, prevention, monitoring, treatment or alleviation of disease;
- diagnosis, monitoring, treatment, alleviation of, or compensation for an injury;

- investigation, replacement, modification, or support of the anatomy, or of a physiological process;
- supporting or sustaining life;
- control of conception;
- disinfection of medical devices;
- providing information for medical or diagnostic purposes by means of in vitro examination of specimens derived from the human body; and

b) which does not achieve its primary intended action in or on the human body by pharmacological, immunological or metabolic means, but which may be assisted in its intended function by such means.

Medicine: any substance or combination of substances presented as having properties for treating or preventing disease in humans.

Neglected tropical diseases: a group of diseases that affect (almost exclusively) people living in rural parts of developing countries. They often cause life-long disabilities but are not necessarily fatal.

Performance evaluation: review of the performance of a medical device based upon data already available, scientific literature and, where appropriate, laboratory, animal, or clinical investigations.
Physician preference items: implantable items that come in many brands from which a physician can choose, e.g. cardiac stents, pacemakers, orthopaedic implants.

Primary health care: (1) essential health care made accessible at a cost a country and community can afford, with methods that are practical, scientifically sound, and socially acceptable; (2) the first level contact with people taking action to improve health in a community.

Protocols: local tools that set out specifically what should happen, when and by whom in the care process. They can be seen as the local definition of a particular care process derived from a more discretionary guideline. They are tools that assist in quality improvement and reducing inequalities. Protocols reflect local circumstances, and variation will be due to the differing types of local provision.

Post-market surveillance: proactive collection of information on medical devices carried out by the manufacturers after those devices have reached the market.

Public health: a social and political concept aimed at improving health, prolonging life and improving the quality of life among whole populations through health promotion, disease prevention, and other forms of health intervention.

Research and development (R&D): creative work undertaken on a systematic basis in order to increase the stock of knowledge, including knowledge of humans, culture and society, and the use of this stock of knowledge to devise new items, applications, etc.

Risk: combination of the probability of occurrence of harm and the severity of that harm.

Secondary health care (see also primary/tertiary health care) : specialized ambulatory medical services and commonplace hospital care (outpatient and inpatient services). Access is often via referral from primary health care services.

Telehealth: the use of electronic information and communication technologies to support long-distance clinical health care, patient and professional health-related education, public health, and health administration.

Telemedicine: the delivery of health care services through the use of information and communication technologies in a situation where the actors are not at the same location. The actors can either be two health-care professionals (for example in teleradiology) or a health-care professional and a patient (for example in telemonitoring of patients with diabetes).

Tertiary health care (see also primary/secondary health care): refers to medical and related services of high complexity and usually high cost. Those referred from secondary care for diagnosis and treatment, which is not available in primary and secondary care. Tertiary care is generally only available at national or international referral centres.

YLD (years lived with disability): the component of the DALY that measures lost years of healthy life through living in states of less than full health.

YLL (years of life lost): the component of the DALY that measures years of life lost due to premature mortality.

Annex 1 List of background papers and methods used in preparing the report

List of background papers

Hansen J et al. *A stepwise approach to identify gaps in medical devices (Availability Matrix and survey methodology)* [Background Paper 1 of the Priority Medical Devices project]. Geneva, World Health Organization (http://whqlibdoc.who.int/hq/2010/WHO_HSS_EHT_DIM_10.1_eng.pdf).

Bougie T et al. *Building bridges between diseases, disabilities and assistive devices: linking the GBD, ICF and ISO 9999*. [Background paper 2 of the Priority Medical Devices project]. Geneva, World Health Organization (http://whqlibdoc.who.int/hq/2010/WHO_HSS_EHT_DIM_10.2_eng.pdf).

Tice JA et al. *Clinical evidence for medical devices: regulatory processed focusing on Europe and the United States of America* [Background paper 3 of the Priority Medical Devices project]. Geneva, World Health Organization (http://whqlibdoc.who.int/hq/2010/WHO_HSS_EHT_DIM_10.3_eng.pdf).

Dankelman J et al. *Increasing complexity of medical technology and consequences for training and outcome of care* [Background Paper 4 of the Priority Medical Devices project]. Geneva, World Health Organization (http://whqlibdoc.who.int/hq/2010/WHO_HSS_EHT_DIM_10.4_eng.pdf).

Beenkens F et al. *Context dependancy of medical devices* [Background paper 5 of the Priority Medical Devices project]. Geneva, World Health Organization (http://whqlibdoc.who.int/hq/2010/WHO_HSS_EHT_DIM_10.5_eng.pdf).

Petkova H et al. *Barriers to innovation in the field of medical devices*. [Background paper 6 of the Priority Medical Devices project]. Geneva, World Health Organization (http://whqlibdoc.who.int/hq/2010/WHO_HSS_EHT_DIM_10.6_eng.pdf).

Carlson D et al. *Trends in medical technology and expected impact on public health*. [Background Papre 7 of the Priority Medical Devices project]/ Geneva, World Health Organization (http://whqlibdoc.who.int/hq/2010/WHO_HSS_EHT_DIM_10.7_eng.pdf).

Kaplan w et al. *Future public health needs: commonalities and differences between high- and low- resource settings* [Backgorund Paper 8 of the Priority Medical Devices project]. Geneva, World Health Organization (http://whqlibdoc.who.int/hq/2010/WHO_HSS_EHT_DIM_10.8_eng.pdf).

In 2007, at the request of the Ministry of Health, Welfare and Sport of the Netherlands, the World Health Organization launched the *Priority Medical Devices* project to determine whether medical devices currently on the global market are meeting the needs of health-care providers and patients throughout the world and, if not, to propose remedial action based on sound research. The project was funded entirely by the Government of the Kingdom of the Netherlands.

Literature reviews were preformed to determine the extent to which information was available on medical devices. Based on the preliminary finding of the reviews the project team found it necessary to organize a series of Advisory Group meetings and informal consultations.
The first Advisory Group meeting recommended the Global Burden of Disease (GBD) study as a tool to prioritize the high-burden diseases. For disabilities, a link between comparison between GBD and the International Classification of Functioning, Disability and Health (ICF) had to be made. A literature search and expert opinions should be combined to define the gaps in the availability of medical devices. The experts agreed that the focus of the project should be on medical devices, rather than on health systems.

The Advisory Group was in agreement on the following steps: (1) the general approach of the project (i.e. categorizing medical devices in four categories: preventive, diagnostic, therapeutic, and assistive medical devices), (2) the development of the methodology needed to evaluate these gaps, and (3) the integration of cross-cutting themes in the project.

The Informal consultation provided input on availability and gaps in the field of medical devices, on cross cutting themes and provided input on specific information relevant to the objectives of the project.

Documentation used in this report was on the global burden of disease and disability; on clinical procedures according to guidelines used in the management of diseases; on projections of future disease and disability burdens in the context of demographic trends; on cross-cutting issues such as the training of medical device users, medical device design, on contextual appropriateness of medical devices, on regulatory oversight; and on catalysts of, and barriers to, medical device innovation and research.

A number of background papers were prepared to support the writing of the report (see above).

A Steering Group was formed to guide the writing and to review the report. The Steering Group consisted of experts in the field of medical devices, clinical medicine, regulatory affairs, and from academia. Where reviewer comments conflicted, one or more of the following strategies were used, as appropriate: (1) priority was given to views shared by the majority of reviewers; (2) the text was altered to include both/all views and to detail circumstances where one view might be more acceptable than another; (3) a final decision was sought from additional experts with specific experience in the subject of debate.

Methodology used in the Priority Medical Devices project:
http://whqlibdoc.who.int/hq/2010/WHO_HSS_EHT_DIM_10.10_eng.pdf

Literature review of available clinical evidence for medical devices:
http://whqlibdoc.who.int/hq/2010/WHO_HSS_EHT_DIM_10.11_eng.pdf

Annex 2 Conflict of interest statement

Technical experts who gave input and direction on content from inception to the final stages of the Priority Medical Devices project were asked to confirm their interests, and to provide any additional information relevant to the subject matter.

Steering Group

The Steering Group did not declare any conflict of interest.

Advisory Group

The following interest was declared by a member of the Advisory Group, specifically financial interests related to commercial organizations: Eoin O'Brien is the director of DABL ltd.

Other Members of the Advisory Group declared that they had no conflict of interest in regards to their participation in the project.

Informal consultation

The following interests were declared by members of the Informal consultation, specifically financial interests related to commercial organizations:

Lee Feldman declared having performed consulting activities for Kleiner Perkins Caufield & Byers Impact Instrumentation, Entegrion, GE Europe, International Intellectual Property Institute, Xcellerex, Juvaris, BioProcessors.

Michael Gropp declared being employed and having shares in Medtronic. He also owns shares in Eli Lilly and Company. He is a member of two medical device associations Eucomed (European medical technology industry association) and AdvaMed (Advanced Medical Technology Association).

EDMA (European Diagnostic Manufacturers Association), Advamed, Eucomed and Terumo were present in the Informal consultations as observers.

On the basis of their declared interests in the subject of the meeting and with regard to the nature and extent of financial interests, the above-mentioned participants took no part in the decision-making process.

Eucomed provided comments on the report and these were assessed and evaluated according to the methodology by the Steering Group.

Other participants of the informal consultations did not declare any conflict of interest.

Contributions

The following interests were declared by specialists consulted to provide input, related to commercial organizations:

Kest Huijsman managing director of B.Braun Medical, member of B.Braun Group, Melsungen, Germany and board member of Nefemed, the Dutch Federation of producers,importers and traders of medical devices.

Frank Ruseler, Director sales and marketing, Dutch Ophthalmic Research Center International B.V.

Gijsbert van Wijdeven, co-founder and shareholder Bioneedle Technologies Group B.V.

Annex 3 Steering bodies of the Priority Medical Devices project

Steering Group

David Banta
Former senior researcher with the Netherlands Organization for Applied Scientific Research (TNO) in Leiden, The Netherlands, and Professor Emeritus at the University of Maastricht, The Netherlands

Mitchell D. Feldman
Professor of Medicine, University of California, San Francisco CA, USA

Adham Ismail
Regional Adviser, Health and Biomedical Devices, Division of Health Systems and Services Development, WHO Eastern Mediterranean Regional Office

Carole Longson
Director, Centre for Health Technology Evaluation, National Institute for Health and Clinical Excellence (NICE), Manchester, UK

Eric Mann
Clinical Deputy Director, Division of Ophthalmic, Neurological and Ear, Nose, and Throat Devices, Center for Devices and Radiological Health, Food and Drug Administration, Rockville MD, USA

Les G. Olson
Consultant in Clinical Medicine and Professional Ethics

Jeffrey A. Tice
Assistant Professor of Medicine, Dept of Medicine, University of California, San Francisco CA, USA

Adriana Velazquez Berumen, Clinical biomedical engineer, founder of the National Center for Health Technology Excellence, Ministry of Health, Mexico, and currently with WHO/HSS/EHT/DIM.

Advisory Group

David Banta
Former senior researcher with the Netherlands Organization for Applied Scientific Research (TNO) Leiden, and Professor Emeritus at the University of Maastricht, The Netherlands

Francis Colardyn
Professor, CEO, Ghent University Hospital, Ghent, Belgium

Carole Longson
Director, Centre for Health Technology Evaluation, National Institute for Health and Clinical Excellence (NICE), Manchester, UK

Eoin O'Brien
Professor, Conway Institute of Biomolecular and Biomedical Research, University College Dublin, Ireland

Tim Reed
Health Action International (HAI), The Netherlands

Martine Guillerm, Medecins sans Frontières, Campaign for Access to Essential Medicine, Paris, France
(Replacement for Martine Usdin)

Mariken Stoutmeijer
Ministry of Health, Welfare and Sport, Department of Pharmaceutical Affairs and Medical Technology, The
Hague, The Netherlands

Ambrose Wasunna (deceased)
Professor, Nairobi Hospital, Nairobi, Kenya

David Williams
Professor, Department of Clinical Engineering, University of Liverpool, UK

Informal consultation

Helen Alderson
Chief Operating Officer, World Heart Federation, Geneva, Switzerland

Robby Bacchus
The Royal College of Pathologists, London, UK

David Banta
Former senior researcher with the Netherlands Organization for Applied Scientific Research (TNO) Leiden, and
Professor Emeritus at the University of Maastricht, The Netherlands

Joey A.M. Van Boxsel
Netherlands Organization for Applied Scientific Research (TNO), Innovation Policy Group, Leiden, The
Netherlands

Francis Colardyn
Professor, CEO, Ghent University Hospital, Ghent, Belgium

Jie Chen
Professor, Director, Key Lab of Health Tech Assessment, School of Public Health, Fudan University, Shanghai,
China

Catherine Denis
Haute Autorité de Santé, Department of Medical Devices Evaluation, Saint-Denis La Plaine, France

Catherine Farrell
MBS Policy Development Branch, Medical Benefits Division, Department of Health and Ageing, Canberra,
Australia

Lee T. Feldman
Chairman, The Institute for Scientific Policy Analysis, Brevard NC, USA

Mitchell D. Feldman
Faculty Mentoring, Professor of Medicine, University of California, San Francisco CA, USA

Chrystelle Gastaldi-Menager
Ministère de la Santé, de la Jeunesse et des Sports, Direction de la Sécurité Sociale, Paris, France

Christian Hiesse
Professor, Service de Transplantation Adulte et de Soins Intensifs, Groupe Hospitalier Necker Enfants Malades, Paris, France

Maurice Hinsenkamp
Professor, International Society of Orthopaedic Surgery and Traumatology, Erasmus Hospital, Université libre de Bruxelles, Brussels, Belgium

Sabine Hoekstra
Ministry of Health, Welfare and Sport, Department of Pharmaceutical Affairs and Medical Technology, The Hague, The Netherlands

Robinah Kaitiritimba
Uganda National Health Users'/Consumers' Organisation (UNHCO), Kampala, Uganda

Peter Leeflang
Ministry of Health, Welfare and Sport, Department of Pharmaceutical Affairs and Medical Technology, The Hague, The Netherlands

Bert Leufkens
Professor, Dean of Pharmaceutical Sciences, Utrecht University, Faculty of Science, Utrecht, The Netherlands

Carole Longson
Director, Centre for Health Technology Evaluation, National Institute for Health and Clinical Excellence (NICE), Manchester, UK

Claude Manelfe
Professor, President, International Society of Radiology, Bethesda MD, USA

Eric A. Mann
Ear, Nose and Throat Devices Branch, Division of Ophthalmic and Ear, Nose and Throat Devices, U.S. Food and Drug Administration, Rockville MD, USA

Utz P. Merten
Yellow Fever Vaccination Center, Köln, Germany

Chiaki Miyoshi
Assistant Director, Bureau of International Cooperation, International Medical Center of Japan, Tokyo, Japan

Frank A. Painter
Director, Clinical Engineering Program, University of Connecticut. Heath care technology consultant, Technology Management Solutions, LLC, Trumbull CT, USA

Agnette P. Peralta
Director, Bureau of Health Devices and Technology, Department of Health, Manila, The Philippines

Dulce Maria Martinez Pereira
Centro de Control Estatall de Equipos Medicos, Havana, Cuba

Norberto Perico
Mario Negri Institute for Pharmaceutical Research, ISN COMGAN Research Committee, Bergamo, Italy

Dr M.S. Pillay
Deputy Director General of Health, Ministry of Health Malaysia, Putrajaya, Malaysia

Mladen Poluta
Director, Health Technology Management Programme, University of Cape Town, Department of Human Biology, UCT Health Sciences Faculty, Cape Town, South Africa

Mahjoub Bashir Rishi
Director, Medical Services SOH, Ministry of Health, Tripoli, Libyan Arab Jamahiriya

Michèle Roofe
Regional Technical Director, North East Regional Health Authority, Ocho Rios, St Ann, Jamaica

Greg Shaw
International Federation on Ageing, Montreal QC, Canada

Kunchala M. Shyamprasad
Cardiothoracic surgeon, Public health expert, Martin Luther Christian University, New Delhi, India

Henk Stam
Professor, Department of Rehabilitation Medicine, Head and Chairman, Erasmus Medical Center, Rotterdam, The Netherlands

Mariken Stoutmeijer
Ministry of Health, Welfare and Sport, Department of Pharmaceutical Affairs and Medical Technology, The Hague, The Netherlands

Per-Gunnar Svensson
International Hospital Federation, Ferney-Voltaire, France

Yot Teerawattananon
International Health Policy Program, Ministry of Public Health, Health System Reform, Bangkok, Thailand

Jeffrey A. Tice
Assistant Professor of Medicine, Department of Medicine, University of California, San Francisco, CA, USA

Ambrose Wasunna (deceased)
Professor, Nairobi Hospital, Nairobi Hospital, Nairobi, Kenya

Wim Wientjens
Vice President, International Diabetes Federation, Leidschendam, The Netherlands

Bart Wijnberg
Ministry of Health, Welfare and Sport, Department of Pharmaceutical Affairs and Medical Technology, The Hague, The Netherlands

Observers

Michael Gropp, EUCOMED, Medtronic, Minneapolis MN, USA

Hiroaki Kasukawa, General Manager, R&D Planning, Terumo Corporation, Kanagawa, Japan

Jean-François de Lavison, President, EDMA, Mérieux Alliance, Lyon, France

Sarah Smiley, Global Strategy and Analysis, AdvaMed, Washington DC, USA

Denis Sohy, EDMA, Brussels, Belgium

Janet Trunzo, Executive Vice President, Technology and Regulatory Affairs, AdvaMed, Washington DC, USA

Maurice Wagner, Director General, EUCOMED, Belgium

Herb Riband, EUCOMED, Belgium

Round table panel http://www.who.int/medical_devices/access/en/index.html

Michael Gropp
Chair, International Affairs Focus Group EUCOMED. Vice President, Global Regulatory Strategy, Medtronic. Minneapolis MN, USA

Susan Ludgate
Clinical Director (Devices) Medicines and Healthcare Products Regulatory Agency (MHRA), London, UK

Guy Maddern
Professor of Surgery at the University of Adelaide and Director of Surgery at The Queen Elizabeth Hospital, Australia. Chair INAHTA (International Network of Agencies for Health Technology Assessment) 2006–2009

Robert A. Malkin
Professor of the Practice and Director of Engineering World Health, Duke University, Biomedical Engineering Department, Durham NC, USA

Mladen Poluta
Director, Health Technology Management Programme, University of Cape Town, Department of Human Biology, UCT Health Sciences Faculty, Cape Town, South Africa

Contributors

Fernao Beenkens
Delft University, The Netherlands

Theo Bougie
BRT Advies. Echt, The Netherlands

Damian Carlson
ECRI Institute, Plymouth PA, USA

Vivian Coates
Vice President of Information Services and Health Technology Assessment, ECRI Institute, Plymouth PA, USA

Jenny Dankelman
Delft University, The Netherlands

Yvonne Heerkens
Nederlands Paramedisch instituut. Amersfoort, The Netherlands

Rob Hoehn,
Question Pro. Seattle WA, USA

Warren Kaplan
Center for International Health and Development, Boston University School of Public Health, Boston MA, USA

Marijke de Kleijn-de Vrankrijker
WHO Collaborating centre for the Family of International Classifications in the Netherlands. RIVM. Bilthoven, The Netherlands

Annemiek Koster
Consultant-Methodologist. Leiden, The Netherlands

Olugbenga Oyesanmi
ECRI Institute, Plymouth PA, USA

Frank Painter
Clinical Engineering Program, University of Connecticut. Heath care technology consultant, Technology Management Solutions, LLC, Trumbull CT, USA

Hristina Petkova
Scientist, King's College, London, UK

Pieter Stolk
Top Institute Farma, Leiden, The Netherlands

Hans Werner
Consultant –Methodologist. Leiden, The Netherlands

Review of the research agenda

Sube Banerjee
Mental Health and Ageing, Institute of Psychiatry, King's College, London, UK

Arjan van Bergeijk
AMPC International health consultants, The Netherlands

Rens Damen
AMPC International health consultants, The Netherlands

Frank van Doren
Through AMPC International health consultants, The Netherlands

Wessel Eijkman
Through AMPC International health consultants, The Netherlands

Maurice Hinsenkamp
Service Orthopédie – Traumatologie, Hôpital Erasme, Brussels, Belgium

Ann Keeling
International Diabetes Federation (IDF)

Jan Meertens
International Centre for Emergency Techniques (ICET), The Netherlands

Ahmed Meghzifene
International Atomic Energy Agency

Vikram Patel
London School of Hygiene & Tropical Medicine, London, UK

Mark Perkins
Foundation for Innovative New Diagnostics (FIND), Geneva, Switzerland

Frank Ruseler
D.O.R.C., Zuidland, The Netherlands

Thijs Teeling
Holland Health Tech, The Netherlands

Gijsbert van Wijdeven
Bioneedles Group, The Netherlands

Luc de Witte
Hogeschool Zuyd, The Netherlands

Medical device innovation is driven largely by the need for better solutions and for greater technological capabilities, and also by promising ideas, scientific interest and economic concerns.

To better align medical device innovation with public health needs, increased funding and improved infrastructure is necessary. In addition, better networking among stakeholders may help.